F.A.T.E. MAKER

BASED ON A TRUE STORY

Charles Weaver

About the Author

Charles Weaver is passionate about helping people explore and become the best version of themselves by giving them the tools needed to take control of their lives and not allowing others to decide what they should do with their own. He's an entrepreneur and writer based in Austin, Texas, where he lives with his wife. He loves to travel, read, play word games, and explore the world around him.

His father died when he was three years old, leaving his mom, who never remarried, to raise him and his older sister. When she passed away on March 12, 2023, it had a profound effect on his life. This book was written as a hobby in an effort to understand, implement and maintain the information he learned "outside the box." Only after reflecting on the profound impact his mother's attitude had on his life did he decided to publish it.

Martha Weaver was adopted and had no brothers or sisters. When her husband passed unexpectedly, she became the sole breadwinner for her and her two children. While working at Kentucky Fried Chicken, she was able to go back and graduate college as a medical technologist. Though her and her children lived in a humble dwelling, she always made room for battered women to stay with her until they got back on their feet.

About the Book

Becoming a F.A.T.E Maker means taking back control of your life by taking control of your thoughts, and you have to be the one in charge. In this book, I will show you how we can change our long-term fate by taking small steps every day and inspire you to become someone who will never stop dreaming and fighting for what they believe in. We'll see how we can:

- Change the internal monologue we have in order to differentiate between lies and truths, harnessing the power of our brain's capacity for self-improvement and growth.

- Develop intrinsic motivation and create power to combat the force others use to manipulate our actions and progress.

- Understand the concept of regression toward the mean by Peter Keating, acknowledging that extreme outcomes tend to move towards the average over time and avoid making decisions based solely on short- term fluctuations.

- Guard against falling into the trap of the Narrative Fallacy, which leads us to construct overly simplistic and misleading stories to explain complex events and instead seek a deeper understanding of the true causality behind outcomes.

- Learn from Daniel Kahneman's "Thinking, Fast and Slow" to recognize and balance the two modes of thinking in our mind, the intuitive and emotional System 1 and the deliberate and logical System 2, ensuring we make well-informed decisions.

- Be mindful of the Reason Respecting Tendency, which urges us to justify our actions and beliefs based on rational reasons, even if those reasons were not the actual drivers of our decisions.

- Value the importance of seeking Disconfirming Evidence, actively looking for information that challenges our beliefs and hypotheses, promoting intellectual humility, and preventing confirmation bias.

- Acknowledge the influence of Availability Bias, which leads us to rely heavily on information that is easily accessible and readily available, and strive to consider a broader range of perspectives and data.

- Confront "Our Problem with the Narrative," recognizing how societal conditioning and conformity have constrained our aspirations and ambitions, and proactively break free from these limitations to reclaim our dreams and pursue a fulfilling life.

Table Of Contents

Chapter 1:

We're In Control Of Our Destiny Over Time

"Progress is best made in bite-sized steps, just like savoring a favorite meal one bite at a time."

~ Charles Weaver

How would you feel if, before your 2nd birthday, you contracted an illness that left you both deaf and blind, living in darkness and silence, unable to comprehend or make sense of your surroundings? Would you end up writing 14 books and over 475 speeches? Suppose you contracted infantile paralysis at the age of 5, leaving you unable to walk. Would you become the first American woman to win three track-and- field gold medals in a single Olympics and the first African American female to eat at the governor's table in her home state versus serving it? Suppose you were growing up in Venezuela and told to leave after signing in at your first major league baseball tryout because you were too short (5'5 140 LBS). Would you later become the shortest active baseball player in Major League Baseball, hold the all-time record for home runs in the postseason in MLB history, and enter the MLB Hall of Fame? The Sunday Times (London, England) ran a story in 2003 about a group of psychologists that interviewed 300 millionaires; 40% were dyslexic. Malcolm Gladwell coined the term "disadvantageous advantages" to address those whose disadvantages strengthen them.

Now that we live in a social media world, I have coined the term "Elephant Head." When we see the world through the eyes of others, it can be detrimental. We see the success, but not the struggle. We see the mess, but not the message. Therefore, when we are in a challenging season, we don't realize in order to get stronger, we have to lift heavier weights.

Just because we are chained to our current environment doesn't mean that it is forever. Instead, it's just a season. We all have blind spots in our psyche, and we don't know what we can achieve until we start, overcome adversity and succeed. The old saying I'll believe it when I see it is wrong. If you don't believe it, you will never see it. That's not something new. It's been that way for 1,000's of years. When we try and don't succeed, we don't fail; we just haven't succeeded yet. Everyone who quits or doesn't try has an "elephant head!"

A baby elephant and a small child have a lot in common. They are both dependent on others to learn how and what they can do. If there is nobody there to teach them the best way, they move forward the only way they know how. The way they were taught by what they observe until they are mature enough to venture out on their own. Also, both can learn that nothing can hold them down if they become excited. Why? Excitement is energy, the same energy that was studied and observed by quantum physicists and neuroscience. This energy can be high (excitement and hope) or low (unbelief and doubt) depending on our thoughts. We aren't in control of everything every day, but over time, we can control our FATE if we know how. The reason most don't know this is because they were born into challenging environments and never learned how to be a FATE maker because nobody around them knew. This is where mentors come into play. 2B1Ask1. If you want to overcome anything, ask someone who has overcome the same situation, and they will know what you don't know yet.

Did you know it has been clinically proven that we can increase strength without moving? Did you know pharmaceutical companies spend 10's of millions of dollars proving that their pill is more effective than someone's mind? That we can become weak or strong depending on what we are thinking about at the time. Focus Attitude Time and Effort is our F.A.T.E., and it can be changed for the better or the worse, depending on how we use it.

"The greater the artist, the greater the doubt. Perfect confidence is granted to the less talented as a consolation prize."

Robert Hughes

We often gain both confidence and doubt from others, and eventually, we have to choose who to believe. One Friday, when I was in high school, my English teacher called me a "blithering idiot" because I got a question on my homework wrong for the 5th day in a row. I believed her and barely graduated high school English my senior year, not because of what she said, but because what she said reinforced what I already felt. While I was in college, I had the same issue. I could not pass basic English because of my lack of confidence in my ability to write. In hindsight, I didn't want others to know I was ignorant, so I didn't put forth any effort. Every semester, I would drop the class because I felt so uncomfortable and ashamed. That was until I was fortunate enough to take Dr. Neil Cameron's class.

The first paper took me 4 hours to write, and it was only 600 words. When I got the paper back, I made an A. My first thought was he saw how ignorant I was, but since I was showing up on time and putting forth my best effort, he was going to pass me. Over the next three papers, I reverted to my old ways and put forth little effort because I thought he liked me and he was going to pass me. Boy, was I wrong!!

The day had come to get our fourth paper back, and the soft-spoken gentleman from Ireland slammed my paper on my desk. With a loud and disgusted voice, he said, "Son, if you want to look dumb, keep that up, but you're a bright writer if you'd only put your mind to it!" The guy next to me looked at me and said he could not believe that the soft- spoken Dr. Cameron had called me dumb. I sat there grinning because that was the first person, other than my mom, who had ever called me bright. I can vividly remember that to this day. He called me bright.

I got **EXCITED** about writing and later that year changed my major to journalism, in which I earned my degree with a 3.5 GPA. What changed? I did not suddenly gain more knowledge. Instead, his encouragement, even though it didn't sound that way to anyone else, excited me so much that I pulled my stake out of the ground. He honestly thought I was bright. And that got me thinking. All along, I thought that I was dumb, perhaps because I didn't believe in myself or that others didn't believe in me. I was like an **IMPOSTER** in every classroom.

Earning my degree wasn't easy on several fronts. Few people, if any, knew I could not afford both college and food. I worked as a busboy at a popular restaurant where I would eat off people's plates before I scraped them into the trash. I tell people that today, and they think it's gross. Let me tell you, when you are hungry, you will eat what is available, and when you are as hungry for achievement, you will do whatever is necessary if you believe it's worth it.

Elephant Head

When I was a kid, my pawpaw brought me to the circus once. It was fascinating, as well as immoral, to watch the animal's tricks. When we were leaving, I remember seeing the elephants lined up, just standing there, not wanting to run away or, better yet, not believing they could run away. What made me afraid was they were tethered by a simple rope to a stake in the ground. They were so massive they could trample the whole crowd with no effort. Yet, they just stood there until a handler loosened the rope when it was either their turn to perform or load up in one of the massive trailers to be taken to the next show. That image left me wondering for years how that is possible. Elephants are among the strongest, most intelligent,

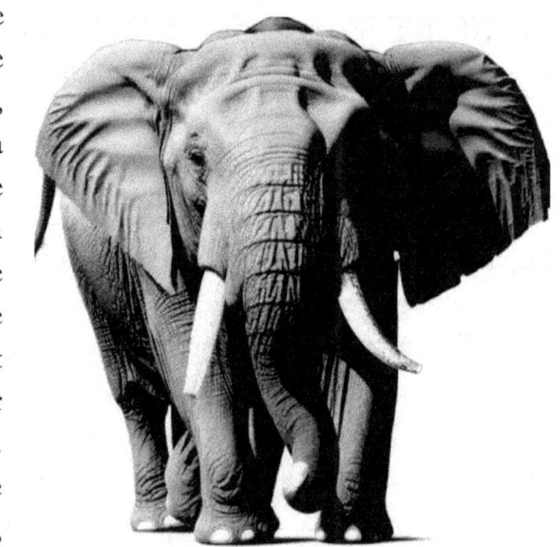

socially intricate, and emotionally complex of non-human species.

Eventually, I started researching and found articles that made me fuming mad that people could be so cruel to such a beautiful creature. These elephants were taken from their mother at the youngest age possible. Then, they were chained to an immovable object until they gave up. Now that they were mature, they "learned" they couldn't get free if tethered. Yet, if they got excited and accidentally yanked the stake out of the ground, they had to be set free because now they learned they were strong enough to break free from anything, and they would never LET anyone tether them again. We all have elephant heads until we don't. Therapists talk about changing the story in our minds, which means the things we replay over and over in our brains. We can replay encouragement or discouragement. It's our choice, and that choice is directly responsible for our F.A.T.E. A baby elephant and a small child have a lot in common. They are both dependent on others to learn how and what they can do. If there is no one there to teach them the best way, they move forward the only way they know how. The way they were taught from what they observed in their environment. Also, both can learn that nothing can hold them down if they become excited. Once we have identified our elephant and see the possibilities, the challenge is staying excited and to avoid becoming victim to the imposter syndrome.

The Impostor Syndrome

In a world filled with high expectations and constant comparisons, impostor syndrome has emerged as a psychological phenomenon that affects individuals from various walks of life. Originating from the field of psychology, the impostor syndrome refers to an internalized fear of being exposed as a fraud despite evidence of competence and success.

Let's explore the imposter syndrome, its underlying causes, its impact on individuals and society, and potential strategies for overcoming it. The impostor syndrome is characterized by persistent feelings of self- doubt, inadequacy, and a fear of being exposed as a fraud despite evidence of accomplishments and competence. Individuals experiencing the impostor syndrome often attribute their successes to luck, timing, or the efforts of others rather than acknowledging their own abilities. This psychological phenomenon was first identified by psychologists Pauline Clance and Suzanne Imes, who studied high-achieving women experiencing self-doubt despite their achievements.

Several factors contribute to the development of the impostor syndrome. One key factor is perfectionism, which often leads individuals to set unrealistic expectations for themselves and fear failure or criticism. Another factor is the fear of evaluation, where individuals worry excessively about judgment from others, leading them to discount their own abilities; social and cultural pressures, such as gender roles or imposter syndrome in minority groups, exacerbate feelings of inadequacy. The impostor syndrome has a negative effect on our health, self-esteem, and well-being. The constant fear of being exposed as a fraud can lead to chronic stress, anxiety, and depression. It also limits individuals' willingness to take on new challenges or pursue their ambitions, as they fear they are not up to the expectations.

Moreover, the impostor syndrome can impair professional growth, as individuals may hesitate to seek promotions or accolades due to a deep-seated belief that they are undeserving of success. The impostor syndrome is not limited to a particular professional background. It can affect individuals across various industries, academia, business, the arts, and sports. For instance, researchers may doubt the significance of their work, business professionals may question their ability to make sound decisions, and artists may struggle with feeling like they are frauds despite the creative talent that others appreciate. Recognizing that the impostor syndrome is widespread can help individuals realize that they are not alone in self-doubt.

While feeling as if we are an impostor, which is doubting we will be able to duplicate our success, there are strategies we can employ to overcome the grip of the imposter syndrome. First, acknowledging and accepting one's accomplishments and abilities is essential. Some of us live in environments that are so critical of people boasting about their talents that we are afraid to acknowledge our own to ourselves. Celebrating achievements and attributing success to personal skills and efforts can help counteract feelings of inadequacy. Seeking support from mentors, counselors, or trusted friends can also provide valuable perspective and reassurance. Additionally, we can alleviate the fear of failure by practicing self-compassion and reminding ourselves that making mistakes is a natural part of growth.

The impostor syndrome is a psychological phenomenon that affects individuals from all walks of life. Personal and professional growth impacts mental well-being. By understanding the underlying causes of the impostor syndrome and employing strategies to overcome it, we can break free from the cycle of self-doubt and embrace our achievements with confidence. Ultimately, by destigmatizing the impostor syndrome and fostering a supportive environment, we can empower ourselves to thrive and reach our full potential. The imposture syndrome is what the world uses to reinforce the fallacious theory that we are born and die in a situation that we have no power to change. The world has romanticized the idea of a "destiny" as being something unavoidable and that we are going to be a product of our environment, just like our family and friends in the neighborhood. We learn this through years of observation and experience while being tied down. This is an elephant head mentality. Fate can be defined as the direction of your destiny. We are the ones who make decisions and take action to get what we want. It doesn't matter where we are born or how we look. That is all on the outside. Our fate is determined by our F.A.T.E.

It's not as farfetched as it seems; sure, we have outliers like Mark Zuckerberg and Michael Dell, who created billion-dollar companies from their college dorms, but 99.9% of people build upon success. It is **F**ocus, **A**ttitude, **T**ime, and **E**ffort, over time, that empowers achievement. The world tells us that we have to get a degree and be able to pass tests to achieve. While we can have a trade or business idea and never get a degree, we do have to pass seemingly arbitrary tests along the way. The tests I'm referring to aren't administered by a teacher in school. Rather, these tests are administered by a teacher called LIFE. The only way to attain success is by learning to adjust our focus, attitude, time, and effort, or we will give up. The television show "Winning the Lottery Ruined My Life" has numerous stories of people who gained wealth by chance and it made life worse. When we are given money, it can be more destructive than not having money at all. I am not suggesting that the definition of success is being wealthy. The most successful you can be in life is happy and peaceful. The second most successful we can be is others knowing we are a compassionate and loving person who does the right thing because it is the right thing to do. The only reason some people's lives aren't worse is because they don't have enough money to support the destructive habits they have acquired over time. They keep or start failing the life test. When people win the lottery, they can afford anything they want, but they haven't built the discipline and habits that support peace and happiness.

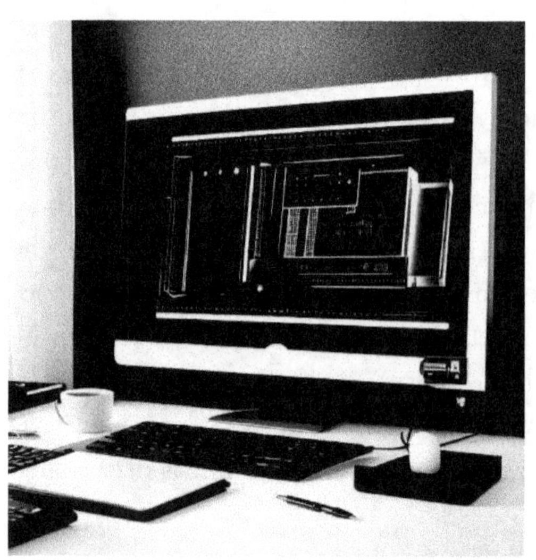

We are in control of our own destiny over time. But that doesn't mean it's going to be easy or glamorous. It takes time to build skills and acquire knowledge. Over time, if you write and execute your plan, you'll find that great things happen, and there is a message in every mess. We also have to make uncomfortable choices and sacrifices. If you want to develop a great business idea and work on it full-time, you might have to quit some of your hobbies and/or hanging out with your friends for a season or two. If you want to drop out of school, be homeless, starve, and beg for spare change to pursue your business idea and/or trade, you can do that, too. You won't be the first and won't be the last. Thousands of people live inside their business until it becomes successful. In fact, immigrants to the United States are four times more likely to become a millionaire than those who were born in the United States, according to author Mark J. Quann. It might be that immigrants often have fewer options and they can't quit. The more options you have, the harder it is to focus and easier it is to quit and try something else. It may also be that immigrants have fewer distractions since they are new to the country and not among all their friends and family. Those who immigrate may also have what Malcolm Gladwell described as a "disadvantageous advantage" versus natural-born US citizens having an "elephant head." Regardless, the seeds of greatness are focus, attitude, time, and effort, and not our last name, the color of our skin, or where we were born.

F.A.T.E. Makers

"FATE Makers ask, seek, and knock."

Charles Weaver

Oprah Winfrey was born into poverty and repeatedly raped as a child by an older family member, according to her podcast, and ran away from home at 13 years old. She was one of 16 African-American students to be integrated into a previously all-white high school until she was sent to live with her father. Then, at 19, she became the first African-American news anchor in Nashville, Tennessee.

Despite all the disadvantages, she became the highest-earning African-American individual in history and is now worth 2.5 billion dollars (Wolfson, 2023). To some, that might be her biggest accomplishment, but not to me. She didn't quit and has inspired millions of disadvantaged children to dream. That alone is worth more than 2.5 billion dollars. Yet, don't get me wrong, if someone tells you they don't care about money, they will lie to you about a lot of other things, too. She EARNED every single penny.

J.K. Rowling was a single mother living in an apartment until she was evicted for not paying rent. Her ex-boyfriend had blown all her money on drugs and alcohol and she had to drop out of school. After a summer of unsuccessfully searching for a job, she had to take welfare and ended up homeless and living off the generosity of friends to eat. Her mother eventually began giving her money to live off of and to go back to school. Still, she could barely survive.

With all that stress on her mind, she took pen to paper and wrote her first book, Harry Potter and the Sorcerer's Stone, in a cafe. She had no idea this was going to be a huge success and a book series, let alone one of the most successful book franchises in history. She got **EXCITED** after reading a book that inspired her to write one of her own. Then it was rejected by 12 publishers. She couldn't quit because she didn't have any other opportunities. The mind is the most powerful tool we have as humans; it can make you feel small and insignificant, or you can turn your problems into assets that help build something bigger than yourself. To achieve greatness, you've got to be willing to go from nothing to something. Our mind is more powerful than any computer and like a computer, it's only as beneficial as what goes into it.

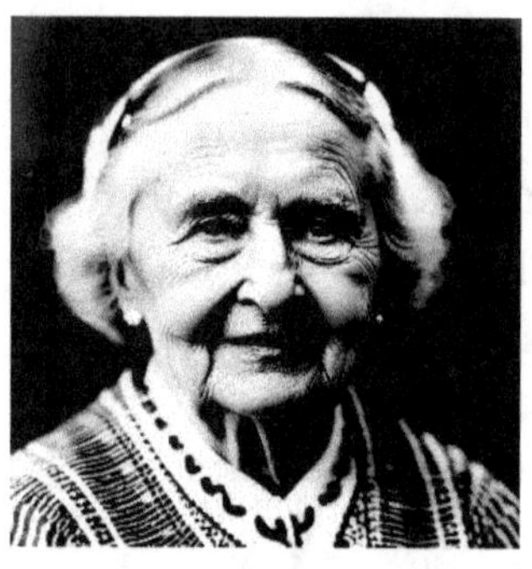

Helen Keller contracted a disease and lost her ability to see and hear before she was two years old. Suddenly deprived of her senses, Keller's world became dark, silent, and scary. Helen's life took a transformative turn when her parents hired a young teacher named Anne Sullivan. Sullivan, herself visually impaired, became Keller's lifeline to the world. She employed a unique method of communication by using her fingers to spell words into Keller's hand, a technique known as finger spelling. Through Sullivan's patient guidance, Keller learned to associate finger movements with objects and concepts, gradually understanding the power of language and communication. She was the **FIRST** deaf-blind person to graduate from college, wrote numerous books, co-founded the American Civil Liberties Union, and was an early supporter of the NAACP.

Speaking to a colleague one day, I told him about Wilma Rudolph in order to encourage him. He responded by telling me he thought about her growing up, but life "took over." I asked him what he meant. He told me about how things hadn't worked out for him for so long that the challenges stole his **FOCUS**. Now, he was constantly thinking about his challenges, which soured his **ATTITUDE**. Now that he had a sour attitude, he had no motivation (**TIME** and **EFFORT**). Things work out best for those who make the best out of how things are working out. The windshield is bigger than the rearview mirror on purpose.

Training salespeople gave me the opportunity to meet a lot of great people. One day, one of my prized pupils comes into the training room. I was so relieved because I had not seen her name in the company bulletin in weeks, and I feared she had resigned. She went on to tell me that she suffers from a rare disease that can make getting out of bed impossible for days and sometimes weeks.

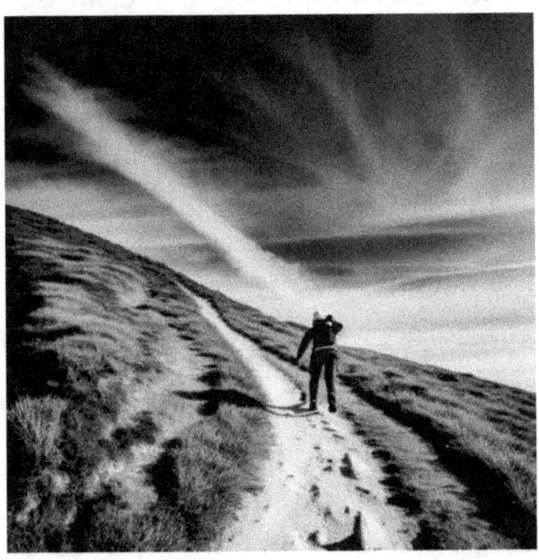

I shall not call her by name because of HIPPA, but she could see the despair on my face. This is when it happened. Quite possibly the most profound and compassionate message I've ever heard. She said, "I don't tell people that to feel sorry for me! I tell people that so they know they are not alone. We are all climbing a hill!" Boom! Drop the mic! That one conversation made me realize we are all dealing with challenges outside of our goals and how we navigate through them determines where we are going.

This was before social media's toxicity had revealed itself. I'm not anti-social media because everything has a good, bad, and ugly side. Yet, today, more than ever, we need to remember we are not alone in our fight and that everyone is climbing a hill, but some hills are steeper than others. That's why we need not forget those who have gone before us and overcome what we are in the process of overcoming.

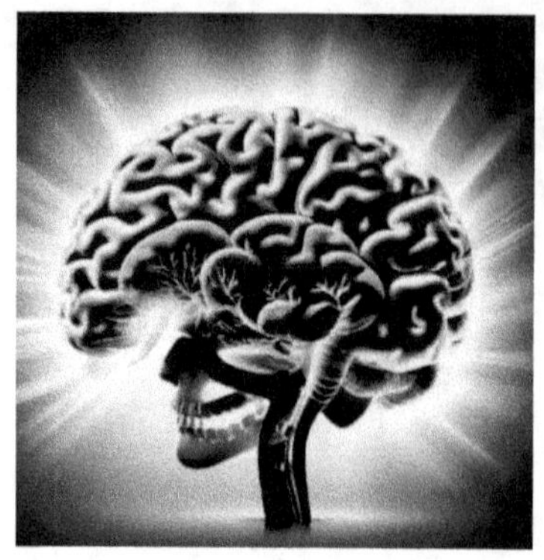

We human beings are more likely to take greater care of our cars than our bodies. The United States' Apollo 11 was the first crewed mission to land on the Moon on July 20, 1969. It was a technological breakthrough, yet it couldn't get off the ground without the right fuel in the tank. What fuel are you putting in your mental tank?

"Our destiny is to fulfill those things upon which you focus most intently. So, choose to keep your focus on that which is truly magnificent, beautiful, uplifting, and joyful. Your life is always moving toward something."

Ralph Marston

The subconscious mind loves finding proof for its ideas and confirmation for its beliefs. When you believe that you're not a public speaker or that people won't be interested in hearing what you have to say, your brain begins to look for proof. It will remind you of that event that took place fifteen years ago when you completely broke down in front of the entire classroom. It will remind you of every single negative comment you've ever heard. People fear public speaking more than death, which means people at a funeral would rather be in the casket than giving the eulogy.

When you think that you're not attractive, your brain will come up with a list of all the things to confirm the belief. You might remember a conversation that you had with a friend earlier this week where they were picking at you about your hair. You might look at that picture on Facebook and get frustrated over how it makes you look. This is your mind trying to reinforce your own beliefs. These are not facts; this is the brain looking for evidence to confirm your opinion. Scientific research concludes that the brain cannot differentiate between a lie and a truth. Your brain will look for proof that your opinions are justified, even if they are proven false countless times.

Psychologists refer to this as confirmation bias (Cherry, 2020), which shows that we are very good at finding evidence to support a conclusion we have already drawn in our mind. If we believe we are not attractive, unable to make a change or not intelligent enough to learn a subject, our mind will set out to look for proof we are right.

Paradoxically, the mind will find proof for all the "positive" beliefs about ourselves, too. When we believe that we're competent, the mind will start searching for proof we are right. It will remind us of every time we were successful at that endeavor. It will remind us of when we went into an interview and nailed it even though all your friends told us that this was going to be a disaster. This is what our mind does, it finds evidence for everything we tell it about ourselves good or bad.

Researchers like Martin Seligman and Mihaly Csikszentmihalyi (Seligman & Csikszentmihalyi, 2000) have done extensive research on happiness and optimal life. They've asked questions about how happy people think, act, feel, and live. And they've discovered an interesting concept they call selective amnesia. When something good happens, we tend to focus on it. We laugh at the funny moments, celebrate the good times, and relish life's successes. In a day or two, the good memories begin to fade, and soon, they'll be gone forever unless we are reminded. When something bad happens, though, it sticks around for a much longer period of time. We remember the bad times and can't seem to let them go. The sadness, hurt, and pain seem to be much more impactful and long-lasting. It is effortless to reminisce about the negative moments, while it takes **EFFORT** to start **FOCUSING** on the positive aspects of our life.

Why does our brain create selective amnesia for positive things, but enjoys dwelling on bad experiences? Why do we romanticize and concentrate on all things negative? We could blame a phenomenon hardwired into our brains: Negativity bias (Nikolopoulou, 2023), which is the tendency to take an overly pessimistic view of future life events. This is a hardwired evolutionary trait, much like our hardwired fear of snakes and spiders. Research has shown that this bias is actually a protective mechanism. It's a way of having us stay in the "comfort zone" where we won't risk physical or emotional harm.

Yet, we're not cavemen anymore. Evolution has changed since the times when we lived in caves; there are no predators looking for us or poisonous plants to eat accidentally. Our world is different, so our minds should be different, too. There's no need to remember the bad times; life has already taught us the things that don't work; all we have to do is learn from them and move on. Keep in mind that the subconscious is always looking for proof that our opinions of ourselves and others are true. The subconscious is always working. How many times have you failed to recall the name of someone or something, and hours later, boom, it comes to the forefront of your mind even though you have been engaged in another activity for hours? While we cannot turn off the subconscious mind, we can take advantage of its power.

Physically writing goals is the easiest brain hack. According to Banu Akgul, CEO and co-founder of ConnectoHub, we are 42% more likely to accomplish a goal if we simply write it down. Remember, we can control our fate over time. Ten years from now, 42% adds up to be monumental. There are a few practical reasons why. Writing a goal enhances clarity, focus, and motivation, but it also gets the subconscious working for us. The subconscious will constantly be looking for ways to achieve the goal and be less vulnerable to distractions. Think of it this way. You know where the spoons are in your kitchen drawer. If there was absolutely no light, complete darkness, you could still find a spoon. You may kick a chair and stub your toe. You may cut yourself on a knife in the drawer, but you could find the spoon. Why not just turn the light on?

In 1981, George T. Doran, Arthur Miller, and James Cunningham authored a groundbreaking article titled "There's a S.M.A.R.T. Way to Write Management Goals and Objectives. This article has since become a cornerstone in the field of management, providing a framework for setting goals and objectives that has been widely acknowledged and implemented. The essay aims to critically analyze the key contributions of the article, highlighting its relevance in modern management practices. The S.M.A.R.T. framework proposed by Doran, Miller, and Cunningham offers managers a systematic approach to goal-setting by emphasizing five crucial criteria that goals and objectives should fulfill:

Specific: Goals should be clearly defined and precise, leaving no room for elusiveness. A specific goal provides a clear direction for an individual or team responsible for its achievement.

Measurable: Goals should be quantifiable, enabling managers to track progress and success. Measuring progress helps to identify areas of improvement for individuals or teams towards achieving the outcome.

Achievable: Goals should be realistic and attainable, taking into consideration available resources, skills, and time constraints. Setting unattainable goals can lead to demotivation and decreased productivity.

Relevant: Goals should align with the organization and objectives. A *relevant* goal contributes directly to the overall success and growth of the business, ensuring that efforts are focused on what truly matters.

Time-bound: Goals should have clear *timeframes*. Setting specific timeframes creates a sense of urgency to prioritize tasks, preventing procrastination and ensuring timely achievement.

This article has made significant contributions to the field of management, revolutionizing the way goals and objectives are accomplished. A structured approach that helps managers craft effective goals and monitor their progress. The S.M.A.R.T. framework has become widely adopted by organizations of all sizes and across various industries due to its simplicity, versatility, and proven effectiveness.

Clarity in Goal: The *specific* criterion of the S.M.A.R.T. framework offers managers a clear roadmap for setting goals that are specific and unambiguous. Focusing on specific outcomes, managers can effectively communicate their expectations and ensure alignment among the team.

Improved Accountability: The *measurable* criterion of the S.M.A.R.T. framework allows for objective evaluation of progress, enabling the ability to hold individuals or teams accountable. This enhances transparency, encourages personal responsibility, and fosters a culture of high performance.

Enhancing Motivation and Engagement: The *achievable* criterion encourages managers to set goals that are within reach, boosting team morale and motivation. Attainable goals provide a sense of accomplishment when achieved, fueling intrinsic motivation towards future targets.

Strategic Alignment: The *relevance* criterion ensures that goals are aligned with the organization's overall strategy and objectives. By linking individual or team goals to the broader organizational vision, the

S.M.A.R.T framework promotes a unified approach to goal-setting throughout the company.

Time Management: The *time-bound* criterion emphasizes the importance of setting deadlines. This helps managers and employees prioritize activities, allocate resources effectively, and avoid wastage of time and effort.

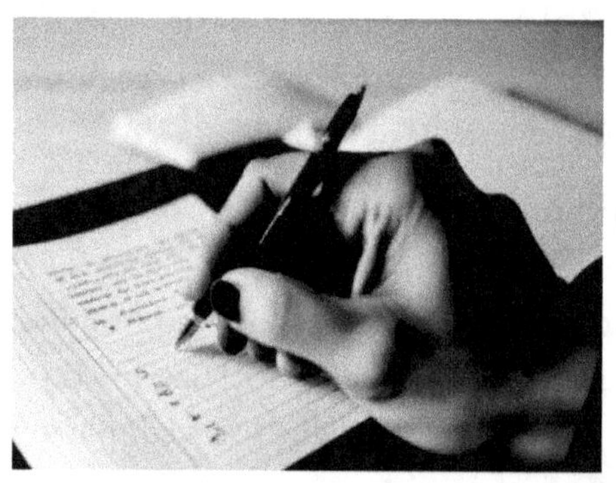

Application and adaptation of the S.M.A.R.T. framework since its inception has evolved and been adapted to meet the specific needs of individuals and companies. Several variations of the original framework have emerged, such as the addition of an "E" for Evaluated or Ethical considerations or the use of different terminology. These adaptations highlight the flexibility and practicality of the S.M.A.R.T. approach in various organizational settings. Furthermore, the S.M.A.R.T. framework has been integrated into performance management and personal development. The versatile nature enables managers to use it at different levels of the organization, from individual employee goals to departmental targets and overarching strategic initiatives.

The 1981 article by Doran, Miller, and Cunningham on the S.M.A.R.T. way of writing management goals and objectives has had a profound impact on the field of management. The simple yet powerful framework has become a widely accepted and implemented approach for goal- setting in organizations worldwide. By highlighting the importance of specificity, measurability, achievability, relevance, and time-bound aspects of goals, the S.M.A.R.T. framework provides managers with an effective roadmap to success. As businesses continue to evolve, the enduring relevance of this article serves as a testament to its enduring value in the field of management.

"If you can't see it, you can't be it. It's just having those brilliant women break out and do something - then other girls can say, I can do it, too!"

Marianne Elliott

Manifestation and The Law of Reversibility

Wallace Delois Wattles' book, *The Science of Getting Rich*, released in 1910 introduces us to the concept of manifestation. He expounded on the universal function of energy as "material from which all things are produced" and emphasized the role of thinking in the manifestation process. When you combine his philosophy with that of Neville Goddard's *Law of Reversibility*, we are given a road map to better understanding the power we have to create the reality we desire, regardless if it is good or bad for us.

The concept of manifestation and the law of reversibility can be better understood with references to scientific principles. For example, just as water can transform into steam and vice versa, circumstances can also produce feelings, and feelings can produce circumstances. This is similar to the principle of mass-energy equivalence, famously expressed in Einstein's equation $E=mc^2$, where E represents energy, M represents mass, and C represents the speed of light.

In the realm of thoughts and emotions, it is important to recognize that thoughts are like waves that carry frequencies and energy. Similarly, mass also carries frequency and energy. However, waves exist beyond the confines of space and time, while mass is bound by them. Therefore, if you can conceive a desire in your mind, it already exists in another dimension within the quantum field, but it lacks mass.

The quantum field encompasses different levels of reality, and although they are distinct, the human mind has the ability to tune into the frequencies associated with each level. Everything in the universe is composed of energy and vibrates at a certain frequency. Thoughts, being waves, significantly influence the reality in which we reside. By combining our thoughts with emotional energy, we provide them with the necessary momentum for manifestation. Emotions, in this context, can be seen as energy in motion. Here, we can draw a parallel with Einstein's equation, where emotions serve as the "light" component. To quantum jump into your desired reality, aligning your vibration with the frequency of your desire is crucial. This is where the power of the subconscious mind comes into play. By consciously controlling your thoughts and emotions, and by reshaping the paradigms embedded in your subconscious mind, you can control your vibration.

It is worth noting that a significant portion of our thoughts are repetitions of what we have already thought in the past. To manifest the desired outcomes, it is imperative to focus our attention and emotions on the thoughts we wish to bring into reality, rather than dwelling on the things we do not wish to manifest. By doing so, we harness the power to consciously reject thoughts that do not align with our desired manifestations and prevent them from materializing into mass.

To further delve into the concept of manifestation and the role of the subconscious mind, it is essential to understand the relationship between thoughts, emotions, and the power of conscious intention. The subconscious mind plays a pivotal role in shaping our reality because it has a significant influence over our thoughts. Many thoughts we have today are simply repetitions of the thoughts we had in the past. This is because the subconscious mind holds and operates based on our ingrained beliefs, values, and programming. To manifest our desires, it is necessary to shift our subconscious paradigms and reprogram our beliefs. This can be achieved through techniques such as visualization, affirmations, and hypnosis. By consciously directing our thoughts and emotions towards the thoughts we want to manifest, we can override previous patterns and create new neural connections in the brain.

However, it is not enough to simply think positive thoughts. Emotions play a fundamental role in the manifestation process. Emotions provide the necessary energy and momentum to attract and manifest our desires. When we align our thoughts with positive emotions such as joy, gratitude, and love, we amplify the vibration and frequency of those thoughts, making them more potent in the quantum field. Conversely, when we dwell on negative thoughts or emotions such as fear, doubt, or anger, we are unintentionally giving energy to those unwanted manifestations. Therefore, it is crucial to consciously reject and redirect such thoughts by focusing on the thoughts that align with our desired reality.

Moreover, the power of conscious intention cannot be overlooked. By setting clear and focused intentions, we direct our energy and attention towards specific outcomes. This intention acts as a guiding force that attracts the necessary opportunities, synchronicities, and resources to manifest our desires.

The science of manifestation (Wattles) encompasses the principles of the law of reversibility (Goddard), mass-energy equivalence (Einstein), and quantum physics (Bohr and Planck). By understanding the relationship between thoughts, emotions, subconscious programming, and conscious

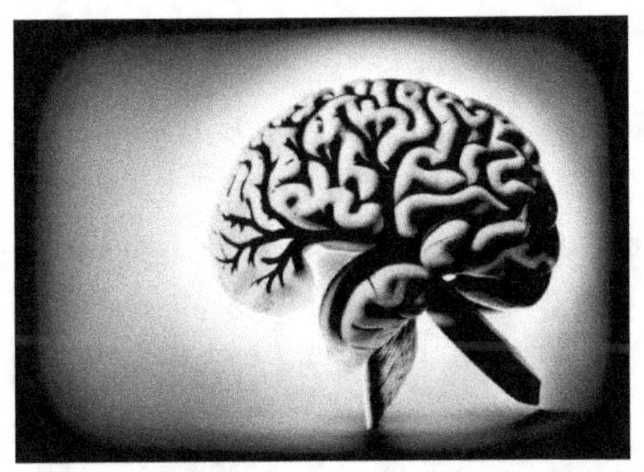

intention, we can harness the power within us to manifest our desired reality. Through thought control, emotional mastery, and aligning our vibration with the frequency of our desires, we can consciously shape our lives and manifest the outcomes we truly seek.

The Law of Reversibility, also known as the Law of Reverse Effect or the Backwards Law, is a principle that describes the connection between our thoughts, feelings, and actions. According to this law, when we act as if we already possess a certain quality or achieved a particular outcome, our thoughts and feelings will begin to align with that action, leading to the manifestation of our desired result. To put it simply, the Law of Reversibility states that by acting in a certain way, we can influence our thoughts and feelings to match that behavior. For example, if we want to become more confident, we can start by behaving confidently, even if we don't feel that way initially. By consistently acting confidently, our thoughts and emotions will eventually catch up, and we will start to feel and think more confidently.

This law is often associated with personal development and self-improvement. It suggests that by deliberately engaging in positive actions, thoughts, and emotions, we can transform our mindset and achieve our desired outcomes. It is important to note that the Law of Reversibility is not a magical solution, but rather a principle based on the understanding of the interconnectedness between our thoughts, feelings, and actions. By consciously applying this law, we can increase our chances of achieving the results we desire.

My wife and I are creatures of habit. Every Fourth of July, we go to the same resort in the Dominican Republic where we were married decades ago. Anibal is our favorite concierge, and we request him every year. We met him on our honeymoon in 2004 while he was working as the "Pepper Cracker." That was his job. He walked around and asked everyone at dinner if they would like fresh cracked pepper. Now, he is the concierge for repeat guests. Thus, he is our concierge. When we visited in 2022, I asked him a question. What do you think about Americans? He told me, "In my opinion, 75% of the Americans who visit here are so stressed and unhappy that it makes me sad. They pay nearly the same to stay here for one week, that I pay for my mortgage for three months. When I first started working here, I thought Americans were mean. Over the years, I realize they are just stressed and unhappy."

When we visited in 2023, I met a psychiatrist from Miami, Florida, while relaxing in the resort pool. He was there with his entire family. Him, his wife, parents, in-laws, three adult children, and their spouses. You could tell he was uber-successful and a true family man. One of his adult children was having a tough time. They had a business that was facing extreme adversity and they were losing faith they could make it successful. I told him about this book. He was understandingly a little aloof about the F.A.T.E. philosophy until I asked him a question. If he were to start hanging out in strip clubs and smoking meth when he returned to Miami, would he still be successful and have a happy family. He looked at me with a grin and simply said, "I see your point. The F.A.T.E. philosophy works both ways. It's like we get out what we put in!"

So, I ask again. How would you feel if, before your 2nd birthday, you contracted an illness that left you both deaf and blind, living in darkness and silence, unable to comprehend or make sense of your surroundings? Would you end up writing 14 books and over 475 speeches? Suppose you contracted infantile paralysis at the age of 5, leaving you unable to walk. Would you become the first American woman to win three track- and-field gold medals in a single Olympics and the first African American female to eat at the governor's table in her home state versus serving it? If you were born with a degenerative spine disease at the age of 4, to a family so poor you often ate cans of dog food, would you play professional baseball? The Sunday Times (London, England) ran a story in 2003 about a group of psychologists that interviewed 300 millionaires, 40 % of whom were dyslexic. Malcolm Gladwell coined the term "disadvantageous advantages" to address those whose disadvantages strengthen them.

THOUGHTS

Chapter 2:

The Physical Power Of Focus

"Where focus goes, energy flows. And where energy flows,
whatever you're focusing on grows. In other words, your life is
controlled by what you focus on. That's why you need to focus
on where you want to go, not on what you fear."

~ Tony Robins

From mental power to muscle power—gaining strength by using the mind (Ranganathan et al 2003) is a fascinating clinical study that found we can increase physical strength without moving. This study was published in JAMA. It is one of the most trusted medical journals in the world. It was performed at The Cleveland Clinic, one of the most trusted research hospitals in the world. The clinicians were actually studying cutting-edge brain imaging technology on volunteers. They placed little probes on the skull of each participant. The probes look like little patches with a wire coming out of them, and the wire goes into a computer. When certain areas of the brain would increase activity, a color would indicate the intensity of the response. The group was split into two so that there was a control measure at baseline. What that means is that each group was tested before the study began so that the clinicians would have a way to measure the results. Then, each group was given a set of instructions that they were to follow every day for the next twelve weeks. This study followed the scientific method rigorously.

The experiment was highly scrutinized and observed and had a p-value of

.005. That means it will repeat itself 995 times out of 1,000. How impressive is that? When a new medication comes to market, medical doctors look for a p-value of .05 before they have total confidence in the studies.

Each individual was given a physical and a battery of other tests before they were picked for the study. The experiment lasted for 5 minutes, five days a week over 12 weeks, involving 30 healthy adults, which, again, were split into two groups of 15. One group was told to sit in a room while the clinicians studied their brain waves after placing the probes on their skulls. That is it. Come in, sit on a chair with these little patches on your head, and we want to study your brain waves to see what this new technology is all about. However, the other group was given instructions to perform a simple mental task while the probes were attached to their skull. Again, this is not an experiment held in science class. This experiment had various control measures to collect data at the end of the study to ensure inconsistent instructions or suggestions did not manipulate the data.

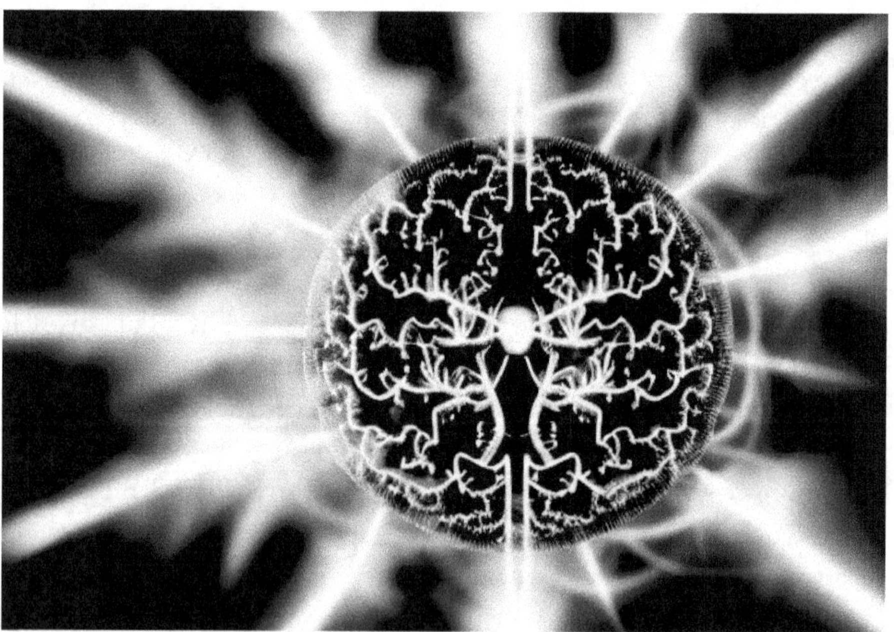

The village idiot can figure out that the group that sat in a chair with this cutting-edge technology placed on their skull will not be the results we will be talking about. The other group was given strict instructions to concentrate on lifting weights with their pinky finger. They were told to envision the weight was getting harder and harder to lift. The clinicians simply instructed them to concentrate on lifting weights with their pinky fingers, but they were never to actually move their pinky fingers. They were to simply sit in the chair and concentrate on moving their pinky finger as if they were lifting heavier and heavier weights.

The clinician's primary objective was to differentiate between a group that was concentrating and a group that was just sitting there thinking random thoughts. Each participant only spent 5 minutes, 5 days a week over a 12-week period, imagining they were lifting heavy weights with their pinky. They were basically meditating on lifting weights.

Once the study ended, the results were astounding. The participants in the group that simply sat in their chairs walked out the same way they walked in regarding the study measures. On the other hand, the group that concentrated on moving their pinky had an average increase of 36% in the strength of that pinky. They never moved the pinky, and they increased strength in actual muscle tissue. They never moved their pinky. Let's build a bigger picture. If that muscle could lift 100 pounds before the study, it could lift 136 pounds after the study, and they never moved the finger.

There are so many things that initiate our thoughts every day that we seldom even realize. What our thoughts are focused on grows, regardless of whether it is good or bad. When we watch a movie, listen to a song, listen to others complaining, we often mentally identify with what we are observing.

What do you think happens when we worry about unpaid bills? It would be great if that would get them paid on time, but what we are really thinking about is why we are having difficulty paying the bills, which increases that difficulty. What happens when you get angry and can't get the cause of the emotion out of your mind? You get more angry right? Well, what if you can focus that same energy on what is going to get better? What if you concentrated on why your relationship is going to get better instead of what is currently wrong? What if you concentrated on the progress you are making toward being great at your job, instead of your boss complaining about something that did not get done the way they wanted? You are already thinking about something, so why not think of improving your quality of life instead of the situation you are in right now? If you are in a great situation, why not think about how it is going to get better instead of the possibility of its decline?

There are those situations we get ourselves into that are the result of our actions and other situations that are due to the actions of others. Either way, what we focus on is going to make the situation better or worse. We can be good at anything that requires mental thought. I cannot jump ten feet high, but I can work ten hours. If you are three feet tall and weigh 50 pounds, you may have limitations that you cannot physically overcome, but there are dreams that you can turn into goals and accomplish by using your F.A.T.E. efficiently.

The study group had one thing on their mind, and that was lifting that pinky finger for five minutes a day, five days a week. What can you accomplish if you get in a quiet place for only five minutes a day and concentrate on why you can accomplish what you desire? The possibilities are endless as long as they are rational. Yet, the rationale all depends on you. Don't let others set your goals for you. Set your own goals and create an environment that will encourage you. Some of us do not have anyone to encourage us. Some of us are in a negative environment. All of us can sit and concentrate on obtaining our goals and desires, but we have to take action. We can't get there until we make steps toward where we want to go.

"When we change the way we look at things, the things we look at change."

Wayne Dyer

When we change the way, we look at things, the things we look at change. When we are focused on the negative, it only makes us focus more on the negative. When we are focused on the positive, we focus more on the positive. Where the focus goes, the energy grows. We can make a positive difference in our lives, but we have to take initiative.

"If a man is called to be a street sweeper, he should sweep streets even as Michelangelo painted, or Beethoven composed music or Shakespeare wrote poetry. He should sweep streets so well that all the hosts of heaven and earth will pause to say, here lived a great street sweeper who did his job well."

Martin Luther King

"Things work out best for those who make the best out of how things are working out."

Coach John Wooden

Celebrate Small Wins

The most rewarding job I've had was working as a sales trainer for one of my mentors, David Morgan. He believed in me and knew that I did the training the way he wanted and not how others or myself felt it should. He started and sold several companies and is one of the most successful people I've ever met. He lived by one motto, "Do It Now." Which encompassed never put anything off, write everything down in a spiral notebook to measure growth, and record three positive experiences in that notebook at the end of every day. He had an entire bookcase that was floor to ceiling of used spiral notebooks with the date he started and ended writing in everyone on the back.

How do you eat an elephant? One bite at a time. Why do you make such small changes in your life? Because they're easy! When we take that first step, the one that starts with "I can do this" or "I believe I can," we move into a completely different mindset. It's like a light switch has been flipped. Life will remind you of everything that is bad. Get a spiral notebook and keep track of everything good that happens. Your brain is keeping score of the adversity. Why not keep a good news journal with things that made you smile, got you excited or you were just grateful for at the end of each day. How do we accomplish goals? By dividing them into bite-sized pieces. The biggest mistake we make is sprinting in a distance race. We start with the most moderate things and work our way up to the bigger and more

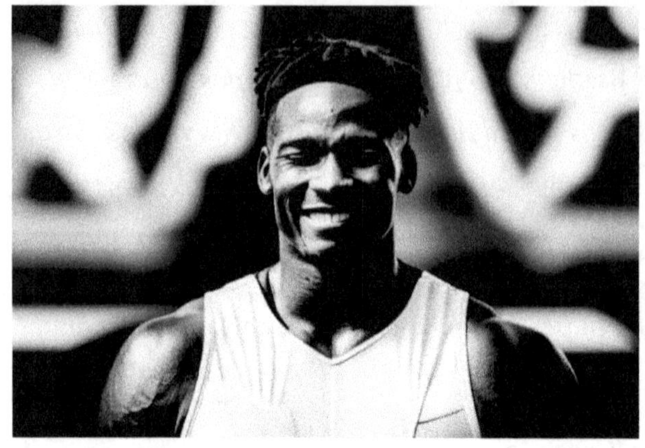

difficult ones. By doing this over time, we get used to achieving these smaller goals and can finally move on to bigger ones. Martin Luther King said it best! You don't have to see the top of the staircase to get there. Just keep taking the next step!"

While playing baseball at a small college, I learned Coach Thorpe's interesting take on goals. Our goal was not to win the small college world series. Our goal was to focus on the things that would put us in the position to win the small college world series. Winning is a reward, not a goal. If you focus on the goal they give you at work, when you get close, you tend to slow down. Once you attain the goal, you coast or quit until the next quarter. However, if daily habits are the goal, you blow the goal out because you keep going. Breaking down goals into pieces works for us in three ways. First, we do not become overwhelmed by such large goals and can face them more easily in smaller units. Second, these small chunks of behavior are easier to remember, which means that you will have more success in sticking with the commitments that you make. Third, this helps us build confidence when we recognize our progress towards a goal. Even the small wins, like getting out of bed in the morning to face another day, are something you should appreciate. Doing so helps to put things in the right perspective and makes us realize how much we have going for us.

It's easy to get focused on the big goals, which will take far longer than you'd like to achieve, but small wins are what keep us going day by day, and it's these that we need to focus our efforts on. You don't have to beat yourself up if you don't manage to do all of your tasks or finish everything that has been set out for you. Keep doing it! Even if the result is incomplete, it will still help you realize that you are doing something productive, and the big wins will eventually happen.

Wilma Rudolph's Determination

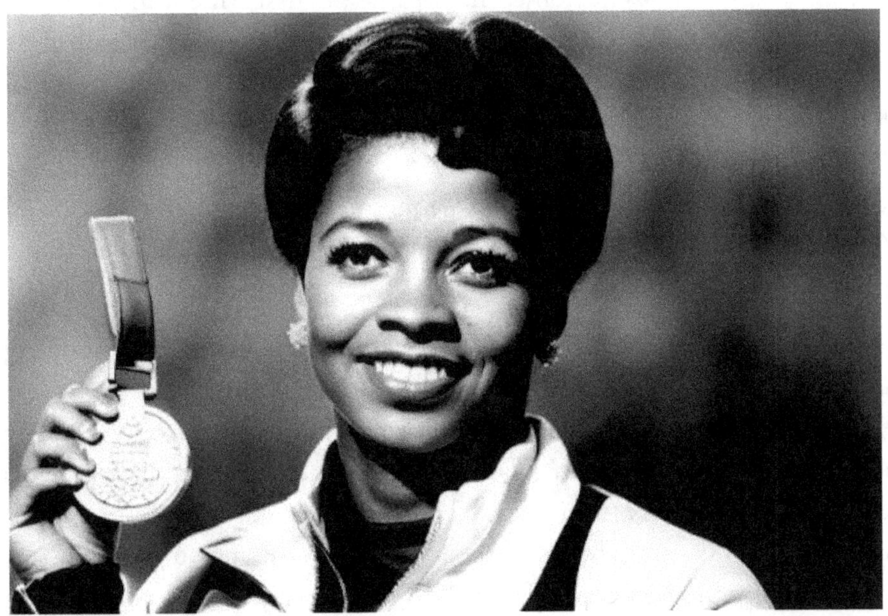

Wilma Rudolph was born prematurely on June 23, 1940, in St. Bethlehem, Tennessee. She faced early health challenges, including double pneumonia, scarlet fever, and polio, which left her with a weakened left leg requiring a brace that the medical community told her she would never be able to walk without. Yet, she would take it off every chance she got to play with her brothers and sisters. Her mother's confidence that she would eventually be able to run and play without it became her own. She didn't know it at the time, but she focused on what she wanted, which was the highest energy. She didn't focus on her problem, she focused on her goal.

When she was twelve years old, she no longer needed a brace or orthopedic shoe to walk. Growing up in the segregated South, Rudolph attended the all-black Burt High School, where she broke records in high school track and field. Her natural talent for running led to her recruitment by Tennessee State University track coach Ed Temple, who recognized her potential and trained her to become a pioneering African-American track and field champion. Despite facing discrimination because of her race, she was selected to represent the United States in the 1956 Olympic Games in Melbourne, Australia. Wilma won a bronze medal at the 1956 Olympics, and she was determined to come back stronger four years later. At the 1960 Olympic Games in Rome, she became the first American woman to win three gold medals in a single Olympic Games, setting world records in the 100m, 200m, and 4 x 100m relay events. When she was informed that her hometown, Clarksville, would be having a parade and ceremony to honor her, she refused to attend unless it was a biracial event. This was the first large gathering that involved people of all races in the history of Clarksville, Tennessee, and the first African-American female to eat at the governor's table instead of serving it.

There's a part of us that believes that we can push past whatever stumbling blocks we face in life and succeed. There's a part of us that believes the impossible is possible. If there's anything that I've learned from legendary athletes like Wilma Rudolph, it is that determination is often the key factor that separates success from failure. Hard work almost always beats talent because talent doesn't always work hard. What we focus on grows. Focus on daily activities and enjoy the wins. Focus on desires and goals. Focus on how badly we want it. Visualize ourself succeeding. A determination that is as strong to accomplish a goal as a starving person's is to eat, or drowning person's is to breathe.

The Brain's Healing Power

Dr. Joe Dispenza experienced a severe cycling accident that resulted in six compressed vertebrae in 1986. Medical professionals informed him that he might never regain the ability to walk and advised him to undergo spinal surgery. However, Dispenza chose a different path. He decided to leave the hospital against medical advice and committed himself to using the power of his mind to reconstruct his vertebrae. Instead of opting for surgery, he employed visualization techniques, picturing each vertebrae healing and visualizing his spine being reconstructed. Astonishingly, within a mere ten and a half weeks, Dr. Joe was able to walk again, and in just twelve weeks, he not only returned to work at his chiropractic clinic, but also resumed his training. This remarkable recovery stands as a testament to the remarkable potential of the human mind.

Dr. Joe Dispenza is an author, lecturer, and researcher known for his work in the field of neuroscience, epigenetics, and the power of the mind. He combines the latest scientific research with ancient wisdom to teach people how to rewire their brains and transform their lives. In his books, Dr. Joe Dispenza explores topics such as the science of change, neuroplasticity, and the mind-body connection. Some of his most popular books include:

Breaking the Habit of Being Yourself: This book delves into the concept of change and how to break free from old patterns and habits that keep us stuck. Dr. Joe Dispenza presents techniques to rewire the brain and create a new reality.

Becoming Supernatural: Here, Dr. Joe Dispenza explores the potential of the human mind and its ability to transcend the limitations of the physical world. He presents scientific evidence and practical tools to tap into our innate supernatural abilities.

You Are the Placebo: This book examines the power of belief and how our thoughts can influence our health and well-being. Dr. Joe Dispenza highlights the placebo effect and provides techniques to harness the mind's healing potential.

In his lectures and workshops, Dr. Joe Dispenza expands on the concepts discussed in his books and provides practical exercises and meditations to help individuals transform their lives. He often talks about the importance of meditation, visualization, and cultivating a positive mindset.

In his book "*Breaking the Habit of Being Yourself,*" Dr. Joe Dispenza explores the concept of breaking free from old patterns and habits that keep us stuck in our current reality. He emphasizes the power of the mind and our ability to consciously create a new and better version of ourselves. Dr. Joe Dispenza explains that our thoughts, beliefs, and emotions shape our reality and influence our behavior. He suggests that many of our habits are deeply ingrained in our subconscious mind and are often based on past experiences and conditioning. These habits can limit our potential and prevent us from creating the life we desire.

To break the habit of being yourself, Dr. Joe Dispenza presents techniques to rewire the brain and create new neural connections. He emphasizes the importance of meditation, visualization, and mindfulness practices to cultivate self-awareness and consciously choose new thoughts, beliefs, and behaviors. Through meditation, individuals can access a state of deep relaxation and tap into the power of their subconscious mind. By visualizing their desired outcomes and embodying the emotions associated with their desired reality, they can create new neural pathways and rewrite the programming of their brains. Dr. Joe Dispenza also emphasizes the role of intention and belief in the process of transformation. He encourages individuals to set clear intentions, believe in their ability to change, and consistently take action aligned with their desired reality.

In his book "*Becoming Supernatural*," Dr. Joe Dispenza explores the potential of the human mind and its ability to transcend the limitations of the physical world. He presents scientific evidence and practical techniques to tap into our innate supernatural abilities. Dr. Joe Dispenza suggests that our thoughts and emotions have a direct impact on our physical bodies and the reality we experience. He explains that by shifting our thoughts and emotions to positive and elevated states, we can activate our innate healing abilities and manifest desired outcomes. One of the key concepts in "Becoming Supernatural" is the idea of accessing a state of coherence between the heart and the brain. Dr. Joe Dispenza explains that when the heart and brain are in a coherent state, they emit a powerful electromagnetic field that can positively influence our health, relationships, and overall well-being. Through meditation and specific practices, Dr. Joe Dispenza teaches individuals how to enter into a state of coherence and connect with the unified field of energy and information. By accessing this field, individuals can tap into limitless possibilities and create profound changes in their lives. Dr. Joe Dispenza also explores the importance of practicing gratitude, cultivating positive emotions, and letting go of limiting beliefs and past traumas. He highlights the role of intention and visualization in manifesting desired outcomes, and provides practical exercises and meditations to help individuals harness their supernatural potential.

In his book "*You Are the Placebo*," Dr. Joe Dispenza explores the power of belief and the influence it has on our health and well-being. He presents scientific evidence and fascinating case studies to demonstrate how our thoughts and beliefs can actually create physiological changes in the body. Dr. Joe Dispenza explains that the placebo effect is a phenomenon where a person experiences a positive outcome or healing response simply because they believe they are receiving a treatment. He delves into the understanding that our thoughts and emotions can produce the same effects as actual physical interventions, such as medication or surgery. In "*You Are the Placebo*," Dr. Joe Dispenza emphasizes that our beliefs and expectations can either limit us or empower us. He suggests that by cultivating positive beliefs and harnessing the power of our mind, we can tap into the body's natural healing abilities and create positive changes in our health. The book explores various techniques, including meditation, visualization, and mindfulness practices, to help individuals harness the placebo effect and activate their body's self-healing mechanisms. Dr. Joe Dispenza also encourages individuals to become aware of their unconscious programming and negative thought patterns, and to consciously choose new empowering beliefs that support their health and well-being. By understanding the placebo effect and the power of our minds, Dr. Joe Dispenza empowers individuals to take an active role in their own healing journey. He suggests that by shifting our beliefs, thoughts, and emotions, we can create profound changes in our physical, mental, and emotional well-being.

Visualization

To a track athlete, the finish line is everything. Our finish line is what we are trying to accomplish. It could be a dream job, a house; it could be my opening an orphanage in Africa. Whatever your finish line is, I want you to visualize yourself as already possessing it.

The difference between a dream and a goal is what we write down. We don't have enough motivation to achieve a goal we are not willing to write down. In her book "*Write It Down and Make It Happen*," Dr. Henriette Klauser explores the profound impact that writing can have on manifesting our dreams and achieving our goals. Dr. Gail Matthews, a psychology professor at Dominican University in California, did a study on goal setting and found that you are 42 percent more likely to achieve your goals just by writing them down.

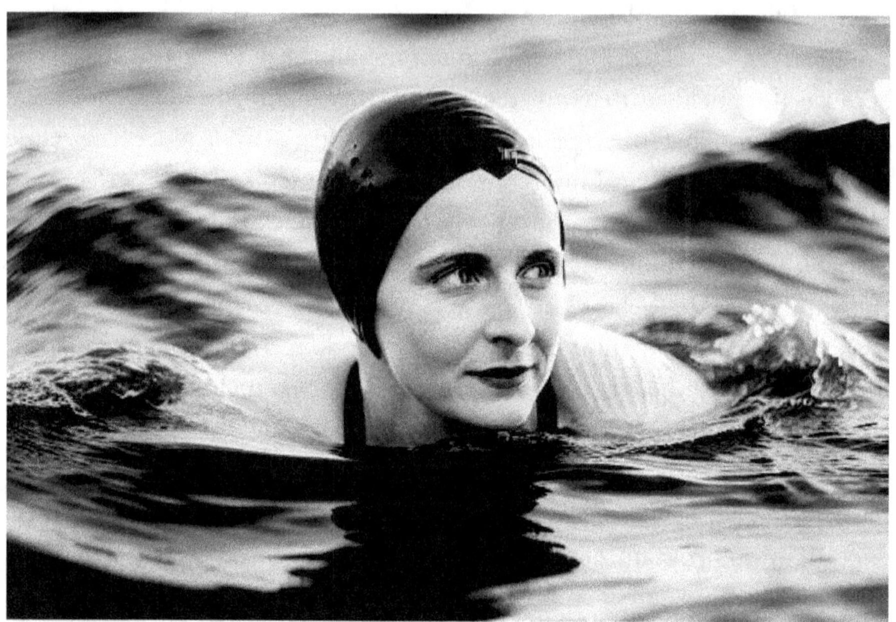

The problem is failure is going to happen. Florence Chadwick was an American distance swimmer who is best known for her world records, like being the first woman to complete the swim between the Catalina Islands and Huntington Beach. The distance between the Catalina Islands and Huntington Beach is approximately 21 miles (34 kilometers) across the Pacific Ocean. She faced several challenges during her swim, including cold water, strong currents, and foggy conditions. Despite these obstacles, she persevered and successfully reached Huntington Beach after roughly 13 hours and 47 minutes. Yet, on her first attempt, she failed. When the fog rolled in, she couldn't see her goal, the beach, and pulled up a short distance from shore. She was asked after she completed the swim how she overcame the same exact obstacles that had caused her failure before. "The first time the fog rolled in, I focused on the fog. This time, when the fog rolled in, I focused on the beach!"

Success is not only about achievement, but dealing with the lack thereof. Ted Williams is widely considered one of the greatest hitters in the history of baseball because he is the only major league baseball player to hit .400 in a season. Yet, he failed 60% of the time. He failed more than he succeeded, but he is the greatest of all time. Failure is going to happen, but to be the best, you have to focus on your success, not your failures.

The invention of the telephone is considered one of the most profitable technological advancements in human history. At the forefront of this groundbreaking invention stands Alexander Graham Bell. Bell's relentless pursuit of his dreams led him to experiment with technologies and concepts related to telecommunication. In the early 1870s, while working as a teacher of the deaf in Boston, Bell began devoting his time to finding a solution to overcome the limitations of existing communication devices.

While determined to make the telephone work, at first, he could not figure out how to make sound waves travel across the wires, even though he had been working with sound waves for a long time. Though he had not given up, he decided put the project aside to work on a telegraph line that would be able to send multiple messages at a time. On March 10, 1876, Bell accidentally turned a screw tighter than before, and he heard a euphonious sound.

He went back to the telephone and, after tightening the same screw from the telegraph, he told his assistant to pick up the listening device on the other end and listen. This is when he successfully transmitted the famous phrase, "Mr. Watson, come here. I want you to," using a device that could transmit and receive speech electronically.

This moment marked a turning point in the history of communication. All along, the device had everything it needed to work, there was just one loose screw. We have everything we need to succeed, but we all have loose screws to tighten. The telephone revolutionized the way people communicated, bridging distances and connecting individuals like never before. Bell's invention had an immeasurable impact on society, transforming the business world, improving personal connections, and inspiring countless future innovations. He faced numerous lawsuits suggesting he stole the technology, but every lawsuit was decided in his favor. See, we all have a loose screw. This may be elephant head, but it also could be a habit, hobby, or even an ideology that is standing in the way of our progress. A lot of times, it's one of these plus an attitude. Think of attitude as a smell because attitudes can compel others or be rejected by others with contempt.

THOUGHTS

Chapter 3:
Physical And Mental Diet

When I was blessed with an opportunity to manage a bar and grill for one of my mentors, Clay Mayeaux, I learned so many valuable lessons talking to the older guys who sat at the bar and ate during their lunch break from work. One day, the president of Northwestern State University, Dr. Chris Maggio, was sitting at the bar eating the daily special. On this particular day, I wasn't feeling too well because I stayed out too late the night before. He noticed and asked when my day started. I told him that I'd been at the restaurant since 9 am. He asked again when my day started. I told him I got up around 8:30 am and came straight to work. Little did I know, while nursing a hangover, I was about to be taught one of the most important lessons anyone could learn.

Dr. Maggio told me he had learned a long time ago that his day didn't start when he woke. It didn't start when he went to bed or the morning before—today started last month. The success he was having today was put into motion last month. His future success was the result of what he did today. He went on to tell me that he knows that someone is lurking in the shadows, preparing, learning, and attaining the experience to outperform him and take his job, and if that happened, it wasn't because of what he didn't do today or yesterday. Instead, it would be due to what he didn't do last month.

We only have to consistently do a little extra to go from ordinary to extraordinary. After all, the only difference is a little extra. This part is not brain science; it's simple math.

Doing the same thing the same way every day! $(1.00)^{365} = 1.00$

Vs

Doing a little extra every day! $(1.01)^{365} = 37.7$

Think of it this way. If I become obese, I can't do it in one day. If I have a heart attack, it's not because of the exercise I missed today or the cholesterol I ingested yesterday. When we don't perform at our optimal level one day a week, after five years, that becomes an entire year. Someone else is working a full day every day, every week, every month, every quarter of every year to get ahead. They will earn your job. That is why everything matters, even the small stuff. Don't sweat the small stuff, but don't ignore it either.

David Hawkins

In David Hawkins' book, Power vs Force, he explains there are two ways of getting things done. First is through force, and I'm not referring to my favorite Star Trek: The Next Generation character, Lieutenant Commander Worf, but rather the use of bulldozing, yelling, and even the occasional use of physical force to get your way. YOU KNOW how we smack the remote when it isn't working properly? That's force.

The other way, according to Hawkins, is through power. Power is an energy described as love in action and is exemplified by luminaries such as

Mother Theresa, Gandhi, or Martin Luther King, Jr. While force is brought by the external, the power that is within us is a drive attribute. The book describes the difference between power and force and how it affects or daily lives. It explains that power is something that comes from within and is based on spiritual principles, while force is something that comes from external sources and is based on fear and intimidation to control. Toxic work environments are led by those who use force. They yell and they undermine those around them to get their way. If you want to succeed at that company, you must do the same. This creates a toxic culture and it's very difficult to right the ship. These are people who are generally promoted to leadership because of a past or present achievement and/or tenure and not because of their leadership skills. According to Laurence J. Peter, author of *The Peter Principle*, everyone will eventually be promoted to a position of incompetence if they stay at a company long enough. What is worse, few organizations will have the integrity to demote them back to a position of competence. On the other hand, leaders that empower us bring out our internal motivation. They don't have to push us to achieve their goal, they empower us to achieve our goal. We have that same power in us to push ourselves, without having to rely on someone else pushing us with force.

There's an energy in each one of us that drives us to achieve the kind of success we want to see in our lives. The key is finding what that energy is and making it work for us. The power vs. Force distinction can be applied to various areas in life: Intrinsic motivation, as we know it, is from within; extrinsic motivation is from outside. Force is different than power. It's externally induced. When we work for a force, we tend to have a day-to-day existence outlook on life because we're always concerned about what people think about our performance or about how they are going to treat us if they don't get their way. This is an energy that comes from outside ourselves, and it's one of the reasons why people take the leap to start their own business. Thy just can't work for incompetent leadership anymore out of principle and/or mental health concerns.

If we want to succeed, we must focus on small goals that will build success over time. This is resilience. When we face adversity, and we will face adversity, we continue the pursuit of the goal in front of us. In the face of adversity, movement toward the goal is extremely empowering because it gives us a reason to keep moving forward. If we are clear about our goals and stay focused on achieving them from within, then our personal power comes through us in the form of action. When our goals are aligned with our spiritual beliefs, we tap into the universe's power. Think about it like this: If we know deep down in our soul that what we want to achieve is right for us, then even when there's a failure or an obstacle in the way, we will persevere and keep moving forward. On the other hand, if our goal is money, fame and power, then we often revert to force.

It's extremely empowering to have the level of confidence that no one can take away from us. When we're not dependent on anyone else for our power and motivation because we create it within ourselves. Our power is our own, and we keep it with us for the rest of our lives. In order to achieve any kind of success in life, there are certain personal traits that must be present: desire, persistence, and belief. We must believe that we can and will accomplish the small goals that build upon themselves. We must have the desire to achieve these goals and the willingness to persevere in the face of all of the adversity we will face.

Mental and Physical Diets

On those "busy" days when we skip breakfast, our productivity seems to take a dip, and we might feel exhausted. The food that we eat has an effect on our mental health and vice versa, but not just because junk food makes us feel sluggish; there's more to it. One of the most studied areas in mental health is the impact of nutrition. Scientific research has shown that certain nutrients are essential for maintaining brain health and can significantly affect mood and cognition. For example, studies have shown that diets rich in omega-3 fatty acids, found in fish and nuts, can lower the risk of depression and anxiety (Matsuoka et al., 2018; Grosso et al., 2014). Additionally, foods containing B vitamins, such as leafy greens, legumes, and whole grains, have been found to reduce the risk of depression and cognitive decline (Skarupski et al., 2010).

In addition to nutrition, certain activities have been shown to improve mental health. Regular exercise, for example, has been found to reduce symptoms of depression and anxiety and improve cognitive function (Lopresti, Hood, & Drummond, 2013; Schuch et al., 2016). Meditation and mindfulness have also been found to have a positive impact on mental health, reducing symptoms of anxiety and depression (Hoge et al., 2013; Khoury et al., 2013). The evidence supports the idea that proper nutrition and regular light physical activity (not lifting weights or running a marathon) can have a significant impact on mental health.

Research has shown that the foods we eat and the activities we engage in can have a significant impact on our mental well-being. Nutrients found in foods such as fish, nuts, leafy greens, legumes, and whole grains have been found to reduce the risk of depression and cognitive decline. Regular exercise, meditation, and mindfulness are also effective in reducing symptoms of anxiety and depression and improving cognitive function. These findings highlight the importance of incorporating healthy habits into our lifestyles to promote good mental health.

If it is challenging to have a good physical diet, it is equally as challenging to have a good mental diet. But it's worth it. We have all heard the phrase "junk in, junk out" when referring to a physical diet. People will count high calories, cholesterol, sodium, sugar, protein, vitamins, etc., to make sure they have a healthy physical diet, but few measure their mental diet. Every action has a thought for an ancestor. There is a growing belief that our thoughts emit certain vibrations that have a profound impact on our mental and physical health. Low- frequency vibrations are associated with negative thoughts, while high- frequency vibrations are associated with positive thoughts. The concept of vibrations is not new to science. Every object in the universe is made up of atoms that vibrate at different frequencies. The frequency of these vibrations determines the energy level of the object. When it comes to human thoughts, the idea is that our emotions and mental states also emit a frequency that can be measured.

Proponents of this theory argue that negative thoughts emit a low-frequency vibration that can have a detrimental effect on our health. These vibrations can lead to stress, anxiety, and depression, which can cause physical health problems such as high blood pressure, heart disease, and immune system dysfunction. On the other hand, positive thoughts emit a high-frequency vibration that can boost our mental and physical health. One study conducted at the University of California, Los Angeles, found that positive emotions were associated with high- frequency brain activity, while negative emotions were associated with low-frequency activity. This suggests that there is a correlation between the frequency of our thoughts and our emotions.

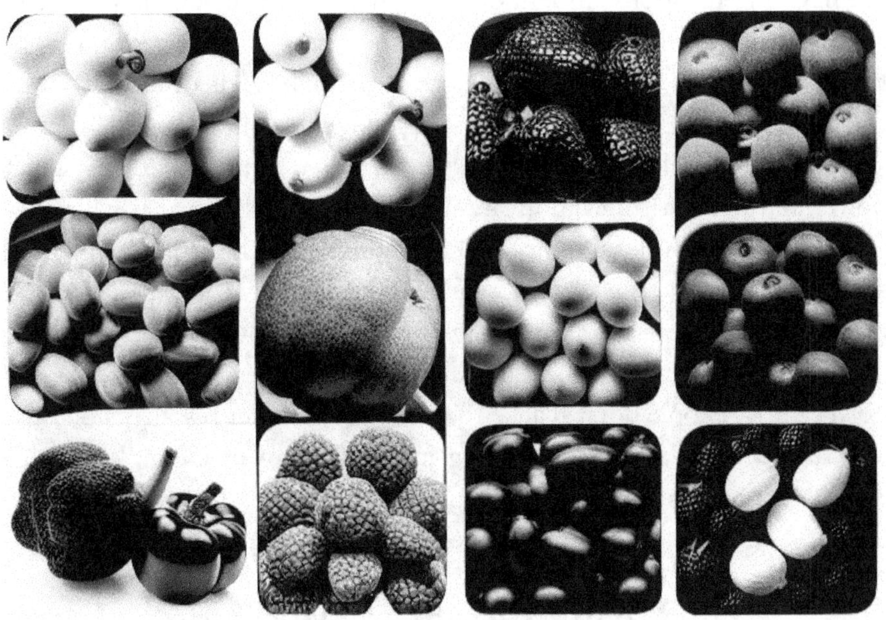

Another study published in the Journal of Alternative and Complementary Medicine examined the effect of sound therapy on the brain. The study found that high-frequency sounds had a calming effect on the brain, while low-frequency sounds had a stimulating effect. This supports the idea that high-frequency vibrations can have a positive effect on our mental and physical health as well.

Our Gut Feeling

When we're referring to a gut feeling, what we mean is trusting your body's instinct over your emotions. Amusingly, the gut DOES talk back to the brain. If you were to observe the vagus nerve, which is the part of the nervous system that connects virtually every major organ in the human body, it would be like a highway through your body. 90% of the traffic would be coming from the gut going to the brain, and only 10% (Glaveski, 2021) would be coming from the brain traveling to the gut. The brain has incredible power, yet through intuition, we can reach even deeper depths of understanding beyond our conscious mind.

We have a tremendous amount of power deep within us that lies dormant and untapped until we are ready to call upon it. And once we do, it's like turning on a light switch that unleashes something inside of us that wasn't there before. This is why so many people love to train for martial arts or any other physical fitness activity, because they can tap into this inner power and use it as their motivation when they work towards what they want—be it weight loss, improving self-confidence, boosting their social skills or anything else. This is why monks spend weeks meditating in mountainous retreats; they are trying to bring their power forth in order to maximize their consciousness and then live their lives from that place of power. Most people don't realize they have these inner resources because they're too busy being swept along in the flow of everyday life. Some people do reach deep inside of themselves and harness their inner power, but most choose not to. How do we tap into our inner power?

The Health Benefits of Meditation

Meditation is a practice that has been used for centuries to achieve a sense of calm, focus, and inner peace. However, in recent years, scientific research has unveiled a multitude of health benefits associated with regular meditation practice. From reducing stress and anxiety to improving sleep and enhancing overall well-being, the positive effects of meditation on physical and mental health are undeniable.

Reducing Stress and Anxiety

One of the most well-known benefits of meditation is its ability to reduce stress and anxiety. When we meditate, we activate the body's relaxation response, which counteracts the physiological effects of stress. Research has shown that the regular practice of meditation can lower the levels of stress hormones, such as cortisol, in the body, leading to a greater sense of calm and peace. A study conducted by the University of Massachusetts Medical School found that participants who underwent an eight-week mindfulness meditation program experienced a significant reduction in anxiety symptoms. Another study published in JAMA Internal Medicine showed that meditation can be as effective as medication in reducing anxiety symptoms in patients with generalized anxiety disorder.

Improving Sleep Quality

In today's fast-paced and hectic world, many individuals struggle with sleep disturbances and insomnia. Meditation has been shown to be an effective tool in improving sleep quality and promoting a restful night's sleep. By calming the mind and slowing down racing thoughts, meditation can help individuals relax and prepare for sleep. A study conducted at the University of Southern California found that mindfulness meditation improved both sleep quality and insomnia symptoms in older adults. Another study published in JAMA Internal Medicine showed that mindfulness meditation can be a useful intervention for individuals suffering from chronic insomnia.

Enhancing Overall Well-being

In addition to reducing stress and improving sleep, meditation has been found to enhance overall well-being. Regular meditation practice can lead to increased self-awareness, self-compassion, and a greater sense of happiness and contentment. Research conducted at the University of Wisconsin-Madison found that individuals who practiced meditation regularly showed increased activity in the prefrontal cortex, the part of the brain associated with positive emotions and well-being. Another study published in the Journal of Behavior Therapy and Experimental Psychiatry showed that mindfulness meditation was effective in reducing symptoms of depression and improving overall psychological well-being.

Meditation is a practice that has been used for centuries to cultivate inner peace, clarity, and mindfulness. While it may seem intimidating to beginners, the process of meditation can be broken down into simple steps that anyone can follow. By incorporating meditation into your daily routine, you can experience the numerous benefits it offers for your physical, mental, and emotional well-being.

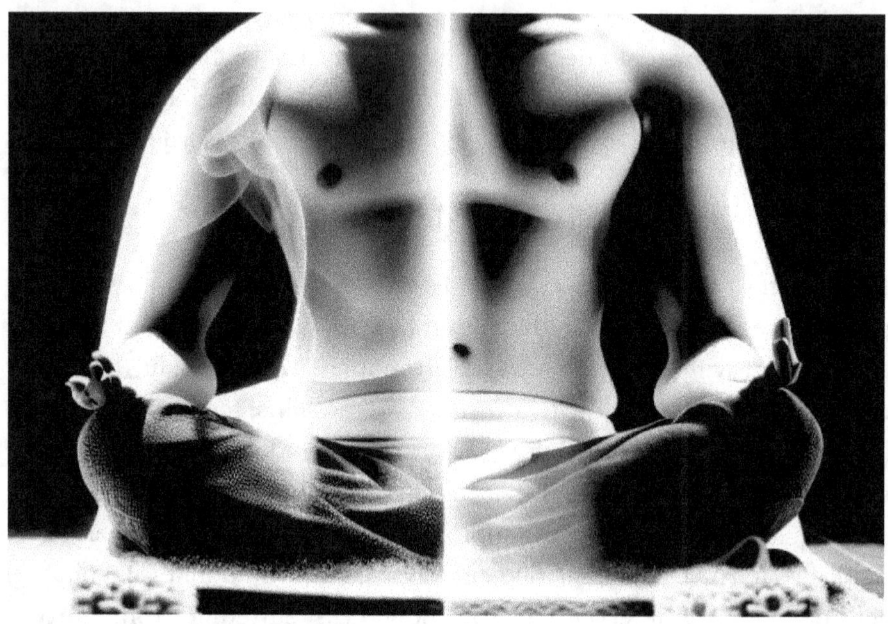

Step 1: Find a Quiet and Comfortable Space

To begin your meditation practice, find a quiet and comfortable space where you can sit undisturbed. It could be a dedicated meditation room, a cozy corner in your home, or even a peaceful spot outdoors. Make sure the space is free from distractions and allows you to relax and focus.

Step 2: Assume a Comfortable Posture

Sit comfortably in a posture that promotes alertness and relaxation. You can sit cross-legged on a cushion, in a chair with your feet on the ground, or even lie down if that is more comfortable for you. The key is to maintain a posture that keeps your spine straight and your body relaxed.

Step 3: Close Your Eyes and Focus on Your Breath

Close your eyes gently and bring your attention to your breath. Notice the sensation of the breath as it enters and leaves your body. You can focus on the rising and falling of your abdomen or the feeling of air passing through your nostrils. Allow your breath to be natural and effortless.

Step 4: Acknowledge and Release Thoughts

As you meditate, thoughts and mental distractions may arise. Instead of getting caught up in them or trying to push them away, simply acknowledge their presence and let them go. Imagine your thoughts as clouds passing by in the sky. Allow them to come and go without judgment or attachment.

Step 5: Cultivate Mindfulness and Present Moment Awareness

Bring your attention back to the present moment by anchoring it in your breath. Notice any sensations, sounds, or emotions that arise in your body and mind. Embrace them with acceptance and non-judgment. Cultivate a sense of mindfulness and present moment awareness.

Step 6: Lengthen and Gradually Increase Your Practice

Start with shorter meditation sessions, such as 5-10 minutes, and gradually increase the duration as your practice deepens. Consistency is more important than duration, so aim for regular daily practice rather than long sporadic sessions. You can use a timer to set the desired duration and avoid checking the time during meditation.

Step 7: Seek Guidance and Support

If you are new to meditation, seeking guidance and support can be beneficial. There are numerous resources available, including books, online courses, and meditation apps, that offer step-by-step instructions and guided meditations. Joining a meditation group or seeking instruction from an experienced teacher can also enhance your practice.

THOUGHTS

Chapter 4:

I Become What I Think

About Most Often

In the 1970s, psychologists Kahneman and Tversky conducted groundbreaking studies on cognitive biases, including the anchor effect. The effect, also known as anchoring bias, is a cognitive bias that influences our decision-making process. It refers to the tendency of individuals to rely too heavily on the first piece of information they are exposed to (the "anchor") when making judgments or estimates.

Consumers may anchor their judgments when comparing products based on their initial exposure to a specific feature or price point. The anchoring effect is a prevalent bias that affects our judgments and decision-making processes. By understanding the underlying mechanisms and being mindful of their presence, we can mitigate the influence of anchoring bias in various domains of our lives. Recognizing the limitations of our initial exposure to information and actively engaging in critical thinking can lead to more balanced and rational decision-making. Anchors can also be influenced by making judgments based on stereotypes or prototypes. Anchor bias can be observed in pricing strategies, where retailers often show higher-priced items before lower-priced items to anchor the consumer's perception of value.

Why is this important? Elephant head! What is the source of your motivation? Is it power, intrinsic motivation coming from within, or is it force, external motivation others use to get you to accomplish their goals? Who or what is the "anchor" of your confidence or the lack thereof? I'm very cautious and weary of negative and/or discouraging people because that is a type of force. Sometimes, we get what we expect and most of the time, a little less, but seldom, if ever, do we get more. We are not a body with a brain. Instead, we are a brain with a body. When we understand the science behind how we make illogical decisions, hopefully, we will be able to make more logical decisions.

Let's look at how pharmaceuticals are cleared by the FDA to be marketed and sold in the United States. Every pharmaceutical that is allowed to be prescribed by doctors in the United States of America has to pass numerous intense studies that are mandated by the Federal Drug Administration. These studies are scrutinized by the FDA, and the findings of the study must repeat themselves in numerous studies and numerous people over numerous years to be approved. These studies cost the pharmaceutical companies hundreds of millions of dollars, and a very low percentage of the drugs that are tested pass the FDA's rigorous testing standards. What is it that each drug must outperform? Another drug? No. Pre-set guidelines for the drug to meet? No. The medication has to outperform the human mind of the person who takes it.

Obviously, before anything can be tested, you have to have something to test it on, and this is where the individuals with certain ailments are recruited. First, there are clinics around the country, and sometimes around the world, that will conduct the studies, and they will begin recruiting the soon-to-be patients. Once there are enough participants recruited for the study, they are divided into groups that are again highly scrutinized. There has to be an equal ratio of race and gender, height and weight, etc. Each soon-to-be patient is informed that they are involved in a study to test the effectiveness of the drug to rid them of the ailment they have been suffering from.

These studies are most often blind in nature. What that means is that both groups know that one group is not actually given the drug in which they are studying. The study is judging if this drug can outperform a placebo, which is as close to nothing as can be created in a pill form. Again, the patients do not know if they are getting the new medication or a placebo pill, but they do know that one group will not receive the real medication. The doctors do not know either. The pills are numbered in the same shape and color. The doctors simply write the number assigned to each pill bottle, and the secret pill police collect the data. There is a predetermined length of time in which the study will take place, and the patients go through a battery of assessments before, during, and after the entire clinical trial. I ask the question again. What does the drug have to outperform? Another pill? No, the human mind. THE HUMAN MIND.

Now, how does the Food and Drug Administration determine whether a pharmaceutical drug actually improves the quality of life of the patients? Well, as mentioned earlier, it must outperform the placebo. What is a placebo pill? A placebo pill is often referred to as a sugar pill. Actually, it is more like a pill made of just powder. The point is that this pill has absolutely no medicinal value. What does medicinal value mean? There isn't any medicine in the pill. As I said, it is only made to look like the pill that is being scrutinized. The patients take this pill for weeks and often months so that the FDA will know if the medication that is being studied is actually significantly more effective at relieving these patients of their ailment than a pill made of powder.

Here is where the tire meets the road, my friend. Some of these patients now have **HOPE**, and hope is the most powerful influence on our thoughts. Every day of their life, for years, they have suffered from something which they could not control. Sometimes, it was physical pain. Sometimes, it was mental illness. Yet, they now have hope and are FOCUSED on how great it is to finally get better. Remember, the mind does not know the difference between a lie and the truth. Therefore, it starts to look for evidence that the hope is well founded. The patient now has a goal to focus on, and they go into the treatment with the intent to feel less pain, have better eye sight, walk straight, and the list goes on and on and on. We are talking about real pain going away. We are talking about real diseases.

This is not a speech to insinuate that everything is pretty and we can go out and tackle the world, and all will be peachy. We are not talking about the path of least resistance, but rather the path where the resistance has the least impact on our ability to keep moving forward when things, people, and stuff are trying to drag us down. Prepare for resistance by preparing a plan to physically change your mental state when life attempts to do it for us. We must have a source to add positive influences and anything that will reinforce our belief that we can achieve our desire. We have to create an environment to combat the environment that is trying, and sometimes purposely, to derail our progress.

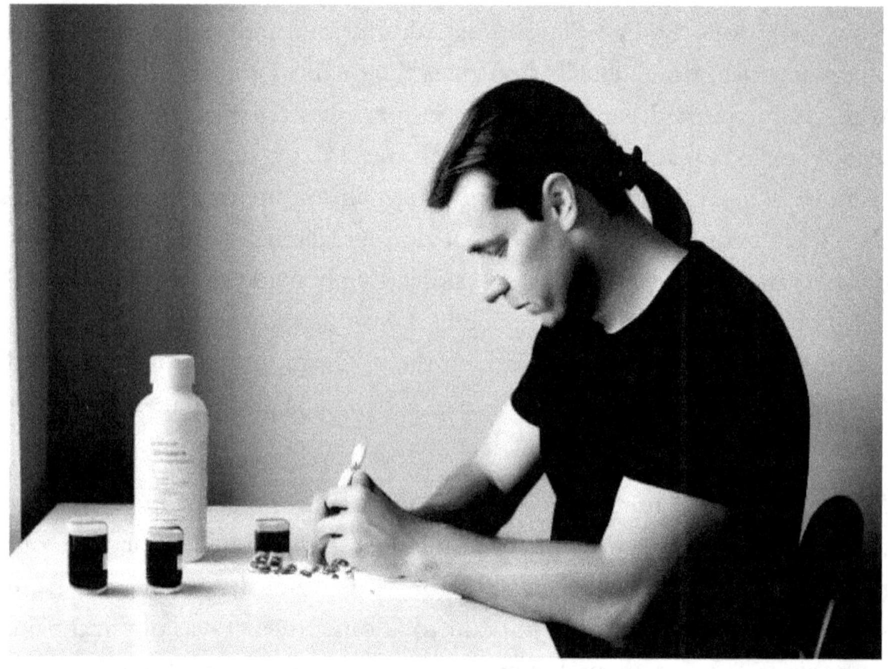

The placebo effect is a fascinating phenomenon in which a person experiences a positive response to a treatment that doesn't actually contain ingredients. In other words, the person's belief in the treatment's effectiveness can cause a physical or psychological improvement. This effect has been observed in numerous studies and can have implications for both medical and psychological treatments. One key aspect of the placebo effect is the importance of expectations (Faith). When a person believes that a treatment will work, their brain can release natural painkillers and other chemicals that can actually help them feel better. This can include reductions in pain, inflammation, and other symptoms.

This physiological phenomenon, where a person experiences a positive response to a treatment that doesn't actually contain active ingredients, can help us achieve success in our lives as well. We can "trick" our brains into believing that we're more confident, more creative, and more successful than we are, and this effect can be harnessed to help us achieve great things. In fact, the phrase, "Fake it till you make it," is a reference to this phenomenon. So, how can we harness the placebo effect? What is the best way to do it?

Positive Affirmations

When we repeat positive affirmations in our minds and consistently reinforce them, our brains begin to believe that we're truly confident and creative even if we aren't. The brain doesn't know the difference between a lie and a truth. It looks for evidence to support what we have told it to believe.

This happens because we begin to mirror the physical responses that someone with confidence would have with their body. So, when you say something like, "I'm so confident I can do anything," and really mean it, as you start to feel more confident, your brain will begin to respond the same way a confident person's brain would. Our brain literally looks for evidence that our thoughts are logical. We can rewire our brains and create new anchors. Some people think this is silly, but if you have the same desire to improve as someone who is drowning and wants to breathe, you have to do a little bit extra. A little extra turns the ordinary into the extraordinary. What you envision yourself being or doing will tend to shape your reality. If you imagine yourself being happy, healthy, positive, and successful in your life, then your brain will look for evidence to support the thought.

Roger Bannister

On May 6th, 1954, Bannister took to the track at Iffley Road in Oxford and, with the help of two other runners, Chris Chataway and Chris Brasher, achieved what many had thought was impossible. You would think that everyone would get excited and encourage Roger. Yet, few people believed he could do it, and most began to discourage his efforts. His peers actually mocked him, and then there were the medical doctors who told him that his heart would beat so fast that he would have a heart attack and die before he finished. Therefore, not only did his peers feel Roger was not fast enough and discouraged his goal, but some medical professionals told him the feat was literally impossible because it would lead to his death. They were not his source. His motivation was from power. Their discouragement was from force.

We, too, sometimes face this same type of adversity when we strive to be the best. In fact, sometimes, the people who love us the most inadvertently discourage our attempts to break the mold. They may feel threatened like Roger's peers, or maybe they feel like others cannot possibly do something they cannot do or won't attempt. Regardless, build a new environment and dare to learn how to combine great effort with a great attitude in all areas of your life.

Roger did more than just distance himself from the naysayers; Roger created an environment. Roger wrote encouraging notes to himself, that others should have been writing to him, and taped them on his bathroom mirror for his own encouragement. When he overheard the taunts of others, he used self-motivators to encourage himself as well. Every time he looked in the mirror, he reminded himself of why and how he was going to achieve his goal. All the while, he trained harder and more often than those he was competing against.

Roger Bannister made history on May 6th, 1954, by becoming the first person to run a mile in under four minutes. Bannister's record-breaking time of 3 minutes and 59.4 seconds was a significant milestone in the history of athletics and one that inspired countless other runners to push themselves to new levels of achievement. This record was one of the shortest records ever held in track and field. Immediately, other track athletes began breaking the 4-minute barrier. What changed in that short period of time? People's brains quit holding them back because they knew for a fact it could be done. Bannister's achievement was not just a physical feat, but a psychological one, too. It shattered the notion that humans had limits to what they could achieve. It also paved the way for others to aim higher and break new records. Since Bannister's historic run, the four-minute mile has been broken by thousands of other runners. What changed? New equipment? It was a mental diet that drove his physical body. Then, others followed because they believed it was possible. Bannister became a neurologist and served as the master of Pembroke College at Oxford University. He was knighted in 1975 for his services to sport and medicine.

We don't pay the price for success. Instead, we pay the price for standing on the side lines and watching others run the race. Run your race one lap at a time, and if you strive to improve upon each lap, you, too, will find yourself in a winner's circle.

Running Your Race

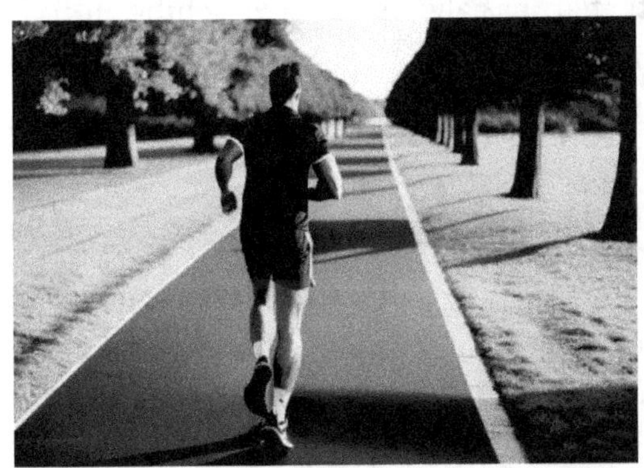

Luckily, we're not Olympic athletes who need to outrun everyone else in the world to win. We don't have to run faster than a speeding bullet or leap buildings in a single bound to win. Who's that person we're supposed to outsmart? The one we were yesterday. Continuous improvement is the difference, and it's what we do best. We have to run faster than our excuses and better than our past. We need to be a runner who will not give up. Now that Bannister has shown us that we don't have to be perfect in order to run this race, he has given us twice the reason why we should better ourselves. It's not about being first or even second in the race. It's about being the best we can possibly be. No matter how many times we fall down, we get back up and continue running. We get up by ourselves because we know that what doesn't kill us only makes us stronger (thanks to Carl Jung).

Have you ever wondered what it means to realize your true potential in life? How can you tap into your inner resources to become the best version of yourself? These are questions that have intrigued humanity for ages, and one person who has deeply explored this topic is Carl Jung, a renowned psychologist and the founder of analytical psychology.

The Collective Unconscious

According to Jung, the collective unconscious of shared experiences, symbols, and inherited archetypes that reside within the depths of our psyche is a reservoir. It is a reservoir of wisdom that transcends time and culture, connecting all humans at a subconscious level. By tapping into the collective unconscious, we can gain access to insights and knowledge that can help us realize our true potential.

For example, let's say you have a burning desire to become an artist, but expectations and self-doubt hold you back. Exploring the collective unconscious, you may discover that art has always played a significant role in history across civilizations and cultures. This realization can give you power, by connecting your goal to something bigger than yourself.

The Process of Individuation

Jung believed that the ultimate goal of human development is individuation. It is the process of becoming aware of and integrating all aspects of our psyche, conscious and unconscious, into a unified, whole self. By embracing and reconciling our inner conflicts, we can achieve a state of wholeness and realize our true potential.

Imagine a person who battles with their own insecurities and fears. They are divided within themselves, torn between their desires and their doubts. Through the process of individuation, they can explore and understand the root causes of their insecurities and gradually integrate and transcend them. This integration allows them to tap into their hidden strengths and talents, ultimately leading to the realization of their true potential and move forward with power without the need to be forced.

Embracing the Shadow

In Jungian psychology, the shadow represents the dark and unconscious side of our personality. It consists of repressed emotions, desires, and traits that we deem unacceptable or undesirable. However, Jung believed that by acknowledging and embracing our shadows, we can unlock immense power and potential.

For instance, let's say you have a tendency to be overly critical of yourself and others. Instead of suppressing or denying this aspect of your personality, I would encourage you to explore the underlying emotions and motivations behind this behavior. By shining a light on yourself, you can see the depth of yourself and work towards transforming them into constructive qualities, such as discernment and empathy.

Practical Steps to Realize Potential

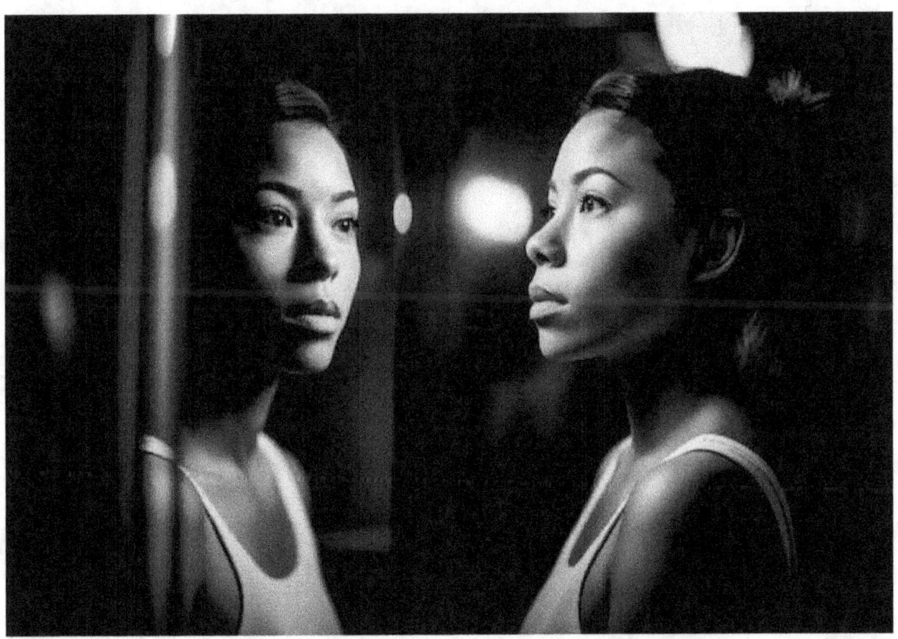

Self-reflection: Take the time to understand yourself better. Reflect on your values, passions, and strengths. Identify any limiting beliefs or fears that may be holding you back from power and pushing you toward the need for force to move forward. Explore the collective unconscious by engaging in activities that deepen your connection with the collective unconscious. This includes studying mythology, exploring symbolism, or engaging in creative pursuits that tap into universal themes.

Embrace your shadows: Acknowledge and accept your shadow side. Engage in shadow work, journaling, or discussing your fears and repressed emotions with a trusted confidant. Use this awareness to transform negative traits into positive qualities.

Set goals: Define clear goals that align with your true potential. Break them down into smaller, achievable steps and take consistent action towards them. Celebrate your progress along the way.

Breaking Personal Records

Motivational speakers love talking about how the comfort zone is where dead dreams are buried, and, in a way, they're right. Always remember, you don't have to beat the records of others to be the best. You only have to beat your own consistently. We get dreams of owning a business, writing a book, having meaningful relationships with our friends and family, regaining our health, and others because our subconscious mind knows that we're capable of achieving them. When we tune into our intrinsic motivation, power, it becomes reality.

Perseverance

Perseverance is the key to accomplishing anything in life. The goal does not matter; what matters is that you decide you are going to do anything and everything it takes to achieve your goal, no matter how long it takes, what it costs, or how big the challenge.

It is said that Thomas Edison made 1,000 attempts to create the light bulb before he finally succeeded. That's perseverance. Do you think we'd have today's comfort of being able to read at night, cook, or take a shower if he gave up the first time he failed? I doubt. Failure is a stepping stone to succcess in that way. It's called perseverance, and it is an extremely useful tool for achieving our goals. People think we have to do so much more to get ahead, and that simply is not true. We only have to consistently, over time, do a little extra to go from ordinary to extraordinary. Again, this part is not brain science; it's simple math. Over time, 1% makes all the difference.

Doing the same thing the same way every day! $(1.00)^{365} = 1.00$

Vs

Doing a little extra every day! $(1.01)^{365} = 37.7$

THOUGHTS

Chapter 5:
The Power Of Attitude

"A wise person can learn more from a fool than a fool can learn from a wise person. Every day, we are one or the other."

~ Bruce Lee

Bruce Lee was a martial artist, actor, and philosopher who is widely considered to be one of the most influential figures in martial arts history. Born in San Francisco, California, Lee spent his early years in Hong Kong before returning to the United States in his late teens to pursue a career in acting and martial arts. One of Lee's most famous quotes is, "A wise person can learn more from a fool than a fool can learn from a wise person. Every day, we are one or the other." Let me ask you a question. If you were an African American born during segregation, with great-grandparents who were freed slaves, you couldn't speak English until you were 10 years old, and never went to school, would you die a multi-millionaire?

The Nocebo Effect: The Dark Side of Belief

When we focus on the positive effects medication can have on our health and well-being, we will improve, and this is called the "placebo effect." The placebo effect, which we read about earlier, has been studied extensively and shown to produce positive outcomes in various medical and psychological conditions. However, the flip side of this phenomenon, known as the nocebo effect, is equally intriguing. The nocebo effect refers to the negative outcomes that can arise from the mere expectation of harm or adverse effects. This phenomenon highlights the significant role that our beliefs and expectations play in shaping our experiences and perceptions of physical and mental well- being. The term "nocebo" is derived from the Latin word "nocere," which means "to harm." The concept of the nocebo effect was first introduced in the field of medical research by Walter Kennedy in the 1960s. Kennedy sought to explore the notion that negative expectations and beliefs could lead to adverse health outcomes, even when no harmful substances or treatments were involved.

The nocebo effect operates through a complex interplay of psychological and physiological mechanisms. Negative beliefs and expectations can activate the body's stress response, leading to the release of stress hormones such as cortisol. This physiological response can heighten pain perception, provoke symptoms, and exacerbate existing health conditions.

Manifestations of the Nocebo Effect

Numerous studies have demonstrated the influence of negative expectations on the experience of adverse effects in various medical treatments. For example, it has shown that patients who are informed about potential side effects of medications are more likely to report experiencing side effects when given placebo treatments. Moreover, the nocebo effect can also impact surgical outcomes. A study conducted by Brody and colleagues (2020) found that patients who were informed about the possibility of postoperative complications reported higher levels of pain and experienced a longer recovery period than those who were not exposed to such information. The nocebo effect is not limited to physical health; it can also affect the course and severity of psychological conditions. For example, in a study exploring the impact of negative expectations on the experience of depression, participants who were given negative information about a fake antidepressant reported higher levels of depressive symptoms compared to those who had been given positive information. Furthermore, the nocebo effect has been observed in the context of psychotherapy. Patients who are informed about the potential side effects of therapy may be more likely to experience negative effects and drop out of treatment prematurely.

Bruce Lee once said, *"A wise person can learn more from a fool than a fool can learn from a wise person. Every day, we are one or the other!"* This quote came to mind after I finished a keynote address, talking about the topics in this very book. A gentleman by the name of Clifton Jolivette told me he wanted to tell me about his dad. I could see the sincerity in his eyes as we walked to a table. We sat, and he began to tell me about his dad, Claude Jolivette. Claude was born in 1908, the grandson of former slaves. His mom and dad didn't speak English. Instead, they spoke Creole, the language of those living on the coast of south Louisiana at the time. They relocated to Houston, Texas, when he was 10 years old.

Claude never went to school because he had to work. Everybody worked, and the earnings went to the household for survival. He learned English while working in a grocery store, where he met a gentleman by the name of Mr. Mike. Mr. Mike owned a gas station nearby and would stop in for groceries several times a week. Over a few years, he and Mr. Mike developed a relationship. He would always comment to Claude's boss about his work ethic and great attitude. One day, Mr. Mike asked him if he wanted to work for him at his gas station. Claude would get a raise and work all the hours he wanted. Well, Claude wasn't working at the grocery store for spending money. The family needed all the money they could get to survive.

Claude went to work for Mr. Mike, and after about 30 days, the business was booming and continued to flourish over the next couple of years. One day, a huge Cadilac pulled up, and the owner of Texaco, Joseph S. Cullinan, got out of the back. Then, the oil companies owned the gas station and leased it out to the person running the business. Texaco had noticed that this one station was not only the top revenue producer in the entire state of Texas, but also outperforming the next four on the list combined. Joe Cullinan offered Mike a job at the corporate office as the head of marketing. The only caveat was he had to duplicate his success at an underperforming station. Then, he would be promoted into the big leagues of oil and gas, opening new stations around the state and eventually the entire country. The only problem was that Mike knew that Claude was the reason the business was booming, not himself. Everyone came to the station because they loved his attitude. Also, Mike could not afford to pay Claude more, even though he would be there by himself for a year. Mike's proposition to Claude was that Claude would get the keys to the place once Mike was promoted.

Claude goes home to tell his parents that Mr. Mike has asked him to do all the work by himself for one year for the same pay and that after one year, he would give him the keys to the business. His parents laughed at how stupid Claude must be to think a white man was going to give a young black man the keys to a business. He was obviously being taken advantage of and that man isn't going to give you the keys. But he did.

After one year Claude was given the keys and Mr. Mike went off to the oil and gas big leagues. The success of the business only increased and eventually, Claude was given the deed and full ownership. Over time, he kept buying the lot next to his. He opened a used car lot. People would sometimes stop paying the note on the car Claude sold them. Clifton would want to go repossess the vehicle, but Claude never let him. His dad would tell him they needed that car to go to work. People would come into the store wanting to buy items and gas on credit. Clifton told him time and again they weren't coming back to pay, and some did not. Yet, every time, Claude would say yes. People would break into the store, and the police would call and ask if he wanted to press charges, but Claude never would. Clifton said he thought his dad was dumb. After all, he never went to school, and they lived in a modest home and drove cars that Claude fixed up.

Clifton confessed that he felt a lot of guilt for thinking his dad was dumb and that the family had no idea how much money Claude had tucked away. Claude always acted like they were broke, yet he always had something to give those who needed it, even when Clifton knew they didn't deserve it. Eventually, the real estate developers came calling, but Claude wouldn't sell. The family could not figure out why. Claude would always tell them they didn't need the money. He told the real estate developers that as soon as he sold out, he would pass, and the money would ruin his kids. Claude ended up selling all the land he had bought, but continued to fix cars until he got sick and passed. He sold his land to the real estate developer who created what is now Memorial Park in Houston, Texas.

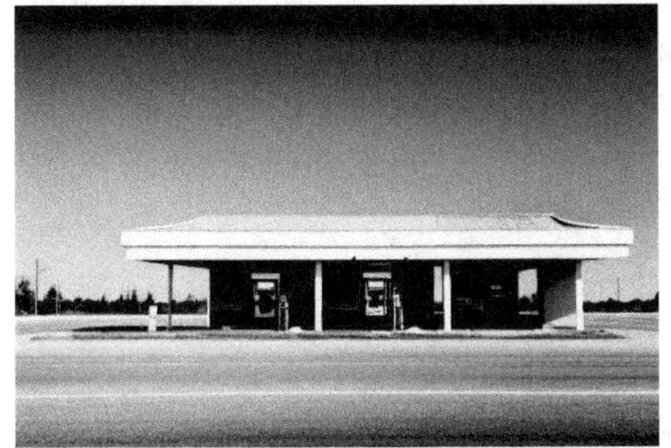

Clifton said, "My dad used to own ALL that land out there." Claude died in 1980, still driving an old truck, wearing oil-stained blue jeans and fingernails that were stained and broken. Though he never learned to read or write, he amassed a fortune of $30 million dollars, and no, the money didn't ruin the kids because, according to Clifton, the man who earned it taught them that it wasn't the most important aspect of their life.

I had tears in my eyes and hair standing up in my arms when Clifton told me the secret to his dad's success. His dad told him, "You can't go broke by giving," and the more he gave, the more God gave him to give. The secret to his dad's success was that God keeps giving to those who keep giving, with a great ATTITUDE. A great attitude was his secret sauce. Claude Jolivette never gave any attention to his negative environment, only the road ahead, and it kept getting better and better.

I cannot imagine someone having more adversity. So, I ask you again. If you were an African American born during segregation, with great-grandparents who were freed slaves, you didn't learn English until you were 10 years old, and never went to school, would you die a multi-millionaire?

What It Takes

Success is subjective. To Warren Buffet, it might mean having a net worth of $100 billion. To others, it might mean being able to take care of family and have time to enjoy life. To Bill Gates, it might mean having a beautiful home and being surrounded by personal assistants. To Bruce Lee, it might have meant being able to train full- time and use his martial arts abilities for good. Whatever definition of success you prescribe, be it material or spiritual, there's a map to discover it. To discover it, it's necessary to go beyond learning what to do and how to do it. Sure, learning the how-to is a critical step, as well as the knowledge you'll need for implementation. The bigger battle is finding out what we are capable of doing, why we are capable of doing it, and a source of power, the intrinsic motivation needed to keep going. Over time, our fate is determined by how we use our Focus, Attitude, Time, and Effort.

Skills?

Skills are learned and built over time, and having the right skills is essential. Skills are like tools in a craftsman's hands; they empower us to apply our knowledge effectively. A skilled individual can transform theoretical knowledge into practical solutions, making them more capable of tackling challenges and achieving their goals.

Knowledge?

Absolutely, knowledge is the foundation of success, but knowledge is gained and built over time. Without knowledge, we lack the understanding and insights required to make informed decisions and take meaningful actions. It shapes our perspectives, broadens our horizons, and enables us to adapt to changing circumstances. Knowledge propels us forward on our journey to success.

Hard Work?

No doubt, hard work, over time, is an essential ingredient of success. Anyone who has achieved greatness in any field will tell you that the long hours of hard work and delayed gratification were a necessary part of achieving their dreams.

As important as these three factors are, they are not sufficient by themselves. The crucial factor that ties all these elements together and elevates them to their highest potential is **ATTITUDE**. If we were to assign numerical values to each letter based on their order in the alphabet, we would have:

A=1, B=2, C=3, D=4, E=5, F=6, G=7, H=8, I=9, J=10, K=11, L=12, M=13, N=14, O=15, P=16, Q=17, R=18, S=19, T=20, U=21, V=22, W=23, X=24, Y=25, Z=26.

Breaking down the numerical values of each word, we find:

Skills

S = 19

K = 11

I = 9

L = 12

L = 12

S = 19

Total: 19 + 11 + 9 + 12 + 12 + 19 = 82

Knowledge

K = 11

N = 14

O = 15

W = 23

L = 12

E = 5

D = 4

G = 7

E = 5

Total: 11 + 14 + 15 + 23 + 12 + 5 + 4 + 7 + 5 = 96

Hard Work

H = 8

A = 1

R = 18

D = 4

W = 23

O = 15

R = 18

K = 11

Total: 8 + 1 + 18 + 4 + 23 + 15 + 18 + 11 = 98

Attitude

A = 1

T = 20

T = 20

I = 9

T = 20

U = 21

D = 4

E = 5

Total: 1 + 20 + 20 + 9 + 20 + 21 + 4 + 5 = 100

Only attitude adds up to 100% because ATTITUDE is the driving force behind everything. It's not a skill or knowledge that can be self-taught from a book or through education at a college. It's not something you can earn, like money or status, either. It's a positive orientation towards life, towards yourself, and towards others that raise our energy to power.

Our Baseline

Though he didn't know it at that time, Francis Galton, in 1886, stumbled across a phenomenon. He noted that exceptionally tall parents seemed to have children who were also tall, but not as tall as their parents. On the other hand, exceptionally short parents tended to have children who were also short, but not as short as the parents. It was almost as if there was a "correcting force" at work, one of nature's mechanisms to offset "extreme" traits in favor of the "norm."

This phenomenon eventually became known as regression to the mean, which is a statistician's way of saying that we tend to return to our "natural" state, though that may not be best for us. While having one hand in fire and the other in ice, on average, we feel pretty good. I get it, but this is more than statistics. Let's look at family income.

The phenomenon is as prevalent in wealth distribution as it is in human height. Regression to the mean is a statistical concept that explains the tendency for extreme observations to move closer to the average over time. In the context of family income, this means that children from high-income families are likely to have incomes that are lower than their parent's income, while children from low-income families are likely to have incomes that are higher than their parents. This brings us back to power vs force. Intrinsic motivation vs external motivation. Some think that factors such as genetic inheritance and environment are the biggest contributors to wealth. While genetics play a role in determining intelligence, skills, and abilities, they do not solely determine an individual's income. Therefore, even if children inherit genetic advantages from their high-income parents, they may not fully capitalize on them when their motivation is from *force*, resulting in lower incomes that regress closer to the mean.

Children growing up in affluent families may have access to better education, resources, and opportunities, but without personal motivation and ambition, they are more likely to be operating with the extrinsic motivation of force, versus the intrinsic motivation of power. Personal faith and ambition are traits from those with intrinsic motivation, power.

Without finding this power, even with a favorable environment, some children may not be equipped to fully exploit them, leading to a regression towards the mean in terms of income. On the other hand, children growing up in underserved families may have less access to better education, resources, and opportunities, but with personal motivation and ambition, traits from those with intrinsic motivation, power, the observations of their incomes compared to their parents will be more extreme.

Regression to the mean emphasizes the importance of individual effort and merit in determining income. While family background and inheritance can play a role, it's the drive that significantly contributes to their income, thus those from underserved families have the same opportunity, but for different reasons. That's why I believe there is hope for us all. It's a mistake to think that you can't be happy or that there are limits to what can be accomplished because of where, who or how we were born. The more enthusiastically we play the hand we've been dealt, the more likely we'll be to win it.

How It Works Daily

When I was a corporate sales trainer, I would call those who had a fast start after training and let them speak to the current class. Normally, you can't get them off the phone; excited salespeople become successful and like to talk. One day, I called Virginia Monceret. Virginia is a great person, wife and mother, but an even better producer. Virginia's performance since the first day she left training was out of this world. She agreed to the call for the benefit of others, and the call was at the end of the day on Friday. This is when a lot of salespeople would take the afternoon to set up appointments for Monday. I called, and she spoke briefly about following the system they were learning in training class. Then she said she had to go. I politely asked why so fast? She said, "Because it seems like every lead I've called this afternoon, I got an appointment." I told her that was great and jokingly said take the rest of the day off. She replied, "I can't. I don't want the NOs to pile up and stop my momentum. I average one appointment for every ten NOs I receive. I know that if I follow the plan, especially while enjoying great success, I will grow vs regressing to the mean. I've got to make the same number of calls regardless of the outcome."

Adversity is unavoidable, but sticking to your business plan limits the probability that you will regress to the mean. When we have a great day and change our routine, our results change over time until we get back to the routine. Every successful business has a business plan. Every business that fails has a bad business plan, quit using the business plan, or never developed a business plan. Without the business plan, regression to the mean is inevitable until it dips below the mean. If your business has thin margins, dipping below the mean can mean instant bankruptcy.

10,000 Hours

The book Outliers by Malcolm Gladwell described how the Beatles were not a good band at first, but they were willing to put in 10,000 hours of practice to achieve mastery (Gladwell, 2008).

Gladwell also talked about Bill Joy, a programmer who learned the limits of computer programming and realized that it could be solved. He then left his job and went on to start his own company, Sun Microsystems, which revolutionized computer technology and made the internet available to the masses.

The thing is that there are no real limits on what we can accomplish in life. This all goes back to the value of persistence. It takes time. If you blow out of the gate, setting the world on fire, you will eventually regress to average unless you have a plan. Yet, even if you start slow, if you follow the plan, you will eventually succeed and increase the mean.

Why 10,000 hours, though? What is it about this number that helps us to achieve mastery? According to Gladwell, this is the number of hours it takes for you to go from a beginner to an expert. We are talking about knowledge and experience acquired over time with multiple repetitions. If we gain success by simply outworking everyone, we will often fall victim to the law of diminishing returns.

Now, what we would like to see is an exponential curve: a fast progression at first when we're getting to know a new skill, followed by a long period of slow growth until we have mastered it and have moved on to the next step. But this seldom happens. Usually, it takes watering the seeds of greatness for a long time before we see the fruits of our labor. This is where 10,000 hours come in. It gives you room to make a lot of mistakes and still make up for them so that you can eventually become a master at what you're doing.

The 18th century French physiocrat, Anne Robert Jacques Turgot wrote about The Law of Diminishing Returns. The Law of Diminishing Returns is a fundamental principle in economics. It helps economists analyze the relationship between inputs and outputs in various economic activities. It is particularly relevant in the context of production, where businesses strive to maximize output while minimizing costs. By understanding diminishing returns, economists can provide insights into productivity, efficiency, and long-term economic growth.

The law of diminishing returns, also known as the law of diminishing marginal returns, is an economic principle that states that as a successive unit of input (such as labor, capital, or resources) is added to a fixed quantity of another input, the overall output or return will eventually decrease. This concept is commonly taught and applied in various fields such as:

Agriculture: Farmers use the law of diminishing returns to determine the optimal amount of fertilizer or irrigation to use on their crops. If too much fertilizer is applied to a field, there may be a point where adding more fertilizer does not increase crop yield proportionally.

Manufacturing: In production processes, companies use the law of diminishing returns to analyze the relationship between inputs (like labor or machinery) and outputs (such as units produced). Adding more labor to a production line may initially increase output, but eventually, the additional workers may result in diminishing returns.

Finance: Investors and financial analysts consider the law of diminishing returns when evaluating investment opportunities. For example, investing more money in a particular asset or portfolio may lead to diminishing marginal returns if the additional investment does not generate proportional additional returns.

Education: The concept of diminishing returns is also relevant in education. For instance, spending more time studying for an exam may initially lead to improved grades, but there may be a point where additional study time does not significantly impact performance.

The point is whatever you want to be great at will take time. Just because you do a lot more, doesn't mean you can beat father time. It means you just keep going. All you can do is all you can do anyway.

We Are What We Think

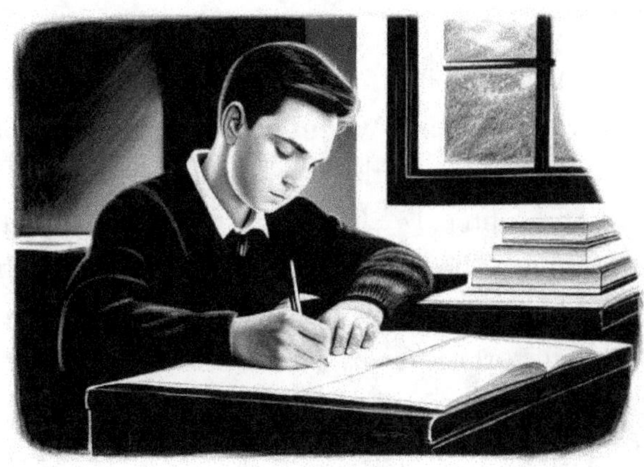

What we feel is what we manifest. We can act like we feel or act like we want to feel. Positive mental attitudes lead to positive results in our life. We can feel our way into a new way of acting or act our way into a new way of feeling. A positive mental attitude (PMA) is a state of mind that enables us to perform at our best because a positive mentality is the fuel that drives those of us operating with intrinsic motivation (power).

Negative, spiteful and aggressive people are operating with extrinsic motivation which is force. PMA is the state of mind that allows us to get excited and getting excited is the only way to break free from elephant head. When we have a positive mental attitude, we feel good about ourselves and we are optimistic about the possibilities in our life that lie ahead. The world is full of opportunities and information, but the only thing that can make a difference in your life long term, is YOU! PMA helps us overcome obstacles; it makes us more efficient, creative, and productive. It enables us to accomplish more than we thought possible and opens the door for leadership and the ability to reach new heights of success and achievement. What's your favorite sport or activity? Do you like doing it? Why? Because it makes you feel good about yourself. It gives your ego a boost. You become involved in whatever it is because you enjoy it. That's a positive mental attitude. A positive mental attitude is like a self-fulfilling prophecy. If you have the right attitude, which is PMA, you believe that things will work out and eventually they do. You act energetically and resourcefully because intrinsic motivation is power and that is the power to make it happen.

When things don't go as planned, do you blame someone or something else? Or do you take responsibility for what happened and try to learn from it so that it will not happen again? When something good happens, do you believe that good things come to those who wait? Or does your thinking go in the direction of this time, I've beaten the odds; this won't last or other negative thoughts? This is the imposter syndrome we talked about earlier. You are achieving, but you are being negatively impacted by people in your life that are motivated extrinsically by others (Force). We can choose how to react to any situation. It's relatively easy to get into a negative mental attitude. For instance, when we are at work and some of our coworkers are goofing off, it is natural to get upset. If you have a negative mental attitude, your responses tend to be negative or angry. The problem, according to the legendary college football coach, Nick Saban, is high achieving people don't like underachieving people and under achieving people don't like high achieving people. Yet, the difference is intrinsic and extrinsic motivation. People who rely on extrinsic motivation often developed what is called *Learned Helplessness*.

Learned Helplessness

Learned helplessness is a psychological phenomenon extensively studied in the field of psychology. It refers to a state of passive resignation or inaction exhibited by individuals who believe their actions have no effect on the outcome of a situation. Learned helplessness was first introduced by psychologists Martin E.P. Seligman and Steven F. Maier in the late 1960s. It emerged from their research on the effects of uncontrollable events on subsequent behavior. Seligman and Maier observed that animals and humans exposed to situations where their actions were consistently ineffective in controlling outcomes tended to exhibit passive and helpless behavior in subsequent situations, even when their actions could make a difference.

According to Seligman, learned helplessness is a result of cognitive processes that occur when an individual perceives that their actions have no impact on the outcome of a situation. This perception leads to the development of a belief that one is powerless and incapable of successfully navigating challenging circumstances. This belief can persist across various domains of life, leading to a general sense of helplessness. Numerous studies have provided empirical evidence for the existence and effects of learned helplessness. In one classic experiment that was horrible and inhumane, dogs were subjected to a series of inescapable electric shocks. Subsequently, when placed in a situation where escape was possible, the dogs exhibited a sense of helplessness and failed to take action to avoid the shocks. Similar findings have been replicated in human studies, demonstrating the generalizability of learned helplessness across species. This is an example of elephant head.

Learned helplessness has important implications for various domains, including education, mental health, and workplace performance. In educational settings, students who experience learned helplessness may become disengaged, believing that their efforts will not yield desired outcomes. This can hinder academic achievement and motivation. In the realm of mental health, learned helplessness has been linked to conditions such as depression and anxiety. Additionally, in the workplace, employees who feel helpless may be less likely to take initiative, affecting their productivity and job satisfaction.

Despite its profound implications, learned helplessness is not an irreversible condition. Interventions and strategies can be implemented to help individuals overcome learned helplessness and promote resilience. Cognitive-behavioral therapy (CBT) has shown promise in treating learned helplessness. CBT aims to challenge and modify negative thought patterns associated with helplessness, empowering individuals to take effective action. Additionally, fostering a supportive and empowering environment can help individuals regain a sense of control and self-efficacy. Learned helplessness can have significant implications for everyday life. Here are a few ways in which it applies:

Personal Relationships: In personal relationships, individuals who have learned helplessness may feel powerless to address conflicts or make changes. They may believe that their actions will not make a difference, leading to a sense of resignation and passivity. Overcoming learned helplessness can help individuals take proactive steps to improve their relationships and address issues constructively.

Workplace Performance: Learned helplessness can impact job performance and career advancement. Employees who feel helpless may be less likely to take on challenging tasks or seek opportunities for growth, limiting their potential. By recognizing and challenging learned helplessness, individuals can develop a sense of self-efficacy, motivation, and take initiative in their work.

Academic Achievement: Learned helplessness can affect academic achievement. Students who believe that their efforts will not lead to success may become disengaged and unmotivated. Overcoming learned helplessness through interventions and strategies can help students regain a sense of control and efficacy, leading to improved academic performance.

Mental Health: Learned helplessness is closely linked to mental health conditions such as depression and anxiety. Individuals who consistently perceive their actions as ineffective may develop a negative cognitive schema that contributes to feelings of hopelessness. Recognizing and addressing learned helplessness can be an important aspect of therapy and self-care, promoting mental well-being.

Goal Pursuit: Learned helplessness can hinder individuals' ability to set and pursue goals. When people believe their actions will not make a difference, they may be less motivated to work towards their aspirations.

By challenging learned helplessness and cultivating a growth mindset, individuals can increase their resilience, persevere through challenges, and achieve their goals.

Overall, learned helplessness has wide-ranging implications for personal growth, relationships, work, education, and mental well-being. Recognizing and addressing learned helplessness can empower individuals to take control, cultivate resilience, and actively engage in shaping their lives. Reversing the psychological impact of learned helplessness requires intentional efforts and strategies. Here are some approaches that can help individuals overcome learned helplessness and regain a sense of control:

Cognitive Restructuring: Cognitive restructuring involves challenging and modifying negative thought patterns associated with helplessness. Identifying and replacing negative beliefs with more realistic and empowering thoughts can help individuals develop a more positive and adaptive mindset. This can be achieved through techniques such as self-reflection, questioning irrational beliefs, and reframing negative thoughts.

Building Self-Efficacy: Developing and strengthening self-efficacy is crucial in overcoming learned helplessness. Individuals can cultivate self-efficacy by setting achievable goals, breaking tasks into smaller steps, and celebrating small successes. Each accomplishment serves as evidence that their actions can make a difference, leading to increased confidence and motivation.

Seeking Social Support: Building a supportive network of friends, family, or mentors can provide encouragement and assistance in overcoming learned helplessness. Sharing experiences, seeking advice, and receiving emotional support from others can foster a sense of empowerment and facilitate the belief that one can overcome challenges.

Taking Action: Taking action, even small steps, is key to breaking the cycle of learned helplessness. By engaging in proactive behavior and actively problem-solving, individuals can regain a sense of control over their circumstances. When faced with challenges, individuals can identify potential solutions, seek help when needed, and take steps towards change.

Learning from Past Successes: Reflecting on past achievements and successes can help individuals challenge learned helplessness. By recognizing instances where their actions made a positive impact or led to desired outcomes, individuals can reframe their beliefs about their ability to influence their circumstances. This reflection serves as a reminder that they have the capacity to overcome challenges and make a difference.

Seeking Professional Help: In cases where learned helplessness significantly affects daily functioning or mental well-being, seeking professional help from a therapist or counselor can be beneficial. Mental health professionals can provide guidance, support, and evidence-based interventions such as cognitive-behavioral therapy (CBT) to help individuals overcome learned helplessness.

It's important to note that reversing the psychological impact of learned helplessness may take time and effort. Each person's journey is unique, and individuals may find different strategies more effective for themselves. By actively challenging learned helplessness and adopting a proactive mindset, individuals can regain a sense of control, resilience, and agency in their lives. Until then they tend to look outside of their current abilities, talents and lives for peace and happiness.

Acres of Diamonds was written by Norman Cromwell. The book talks about a farmer in particular named Ali Hafed. He was a hardworking man who owned a beautiful farm in India. One day, a traveler came to Ali's village and told him stories about precious gems that were incredibly valuable. The traveler spoke of the vast mines in far-off lands where jewels were abundantly found. The tales ignited a spark within Ali, and he became obsessed with the idea of becoming wealthy by discovering diamonds.

Ali couldn't resist the allure of the diamonds, so he sold his farm to embark on a long and arduous journey to fulfill his ambition. Years went by, and Ali's savings dwindled. He had explored countless mines and spent all his wealth, but he never found enough jewels to amount to anything. Disheartened and penniless, he realized that his desire for riches had turned into a nightmare. Filled with regret and sorrow, Ali couldn't bear to face his friends and family empty-handed. He couldn't return because he had sold his farm and had nothing to offer. In despair, he threw himself into the restless waves of the sea and drowned.

Meanwhile, back in Ali's village, the man who had purchased the farm was out tending to the fields. As he was walking along the riverbank, he noticed something sparkling in the water. Curious, he picked it up and realized it was a beautiful diamond. Astonished, he examined his discovery and soon found more diamonds scattered all across Ali Hafed's former farm. As it turned out, the farm Ali had sold to pursue his dreams was, in fact, the largest diamond mine in the entire world. The land was rich with precious gems, just waiting to be unearthed.

We all have acres of diamonds inside of us waiting to be found. The problem is it takes time, and we as humans are generally not patient. Even the sun takes time to come out every day. When a new day starts, it's always dark outside. Even the sun takes time for its light to shine.

The Conversation with Self

I was having a bad day at work one day when Clay Mayeaux, restaurateur and close friend, overheard me calling myself stupid. He asked me to answer a simple question. "If your friends talked to you the way you talk to yourself, would you still consider them a friend?" He went on to say, "Life is hard for everybody, but we don't need everybody in life to believe in us; we just need ourselves, and if there is anyone in your life that talks better about you than you talk to yourself, life is going to be even harder!"

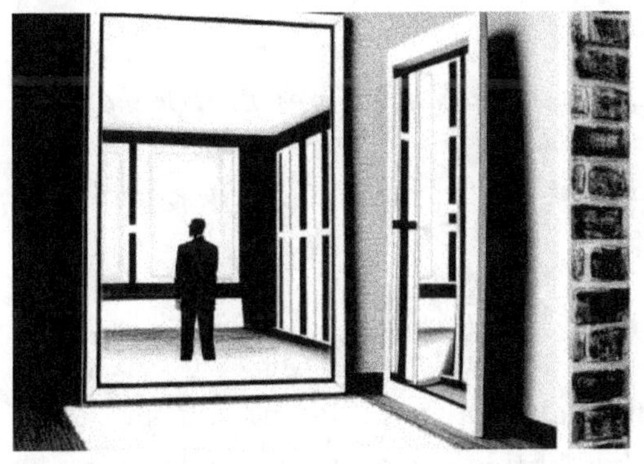

I didn't see it at the time, but that was one of my proverbial loose screws. Just like the one Alexander Graham Bell accidentally tightened too much when he invented the telephone, while making adjustments to the telegraph. Since thoughts influence and often initiate action, thoughts are a big deal, and we are often left alone when it comes to changing that influence in a progressive way. Every action has an ancestor that was a thought.

The person you talk to the most is the "self." Your "self" makes everything happen because your "self" looks for proof that what you are thinking about is true and increases the severity or the progression of your situation.

Adversity + Attitude = Advantageous or Disadvantageous

If you lost both of your parents before you were 15 and your last living grandparent two years later, would you become a successful real estate executive? While directing sales training for a national organization, I met numerous people who made an impact on my life. One of those people is Remy Curry, who is now an uber-successful realtor. She lost both of her parents before she started high school, and her great- grandmother passed when she was 17, leaving her without any guardian. She worked three jobs while earning her degree from Louisiana State University, and we met years later after tragedy had struck again. Now, she was starting over, and after hearing her story, I was left perplexed. See, she had A LOT of reasons to be angry, discouraged and overwhelmed. At least as many as any other person I've ever met. Yet, she beams with positive energy, faith, and compassion. Below is what she wrote me after the training.

Happiness cannot be traveled to, owned, earned, worn, or consumed. Happiness is the spiritual experience of living every minute with love, grace, and gratitude.

Being positive is using your power of choice. Choose to be powerful. Where focus goes, energy flows.

It is not successful people who are grateful. It is grateful people who are successful.

Positive thoughts generate positive feelings and attract positive life experiences.

Remy Curry

The point is that the attitude we choose during our battles with adversity is what determines whether that adversity will be advantageous or disadvantageous. Regardless of whether things are great or bad today, our attitude determines what they will be tomorrow. It's not logical to think someone who had faced so much adversity in her entire life should be so gracious, grateful, and happy. That is what is wrong with the narrative we play in our minds. It is totally logical and expected that any person who moves forward with grace and gratitude will naturally attract success in any and all of their adventures. Attitude is like a smell. It can attract or deter.

While managing Mayeaux's Steak House in Natchitoches, Louisiana, I experienced the opposite. One of the waitresses was about to graduate in accounting: bright smile, attractive, former military, great personality, someone with their entire life ahead of them. Then, one day, she didn't show up for work. It was weird because she was always early and she always asked to stay late. She had taken her own life. That crushed all of us. It didn't matter how we saw her because she didn't see herself that way. Happiness is a choice. Make the right choice when it comes to the way you look at things and the way you talk to yourself. After all, when you change the way you look at things, the things you look at change.

THOUGHTS

Chapter 6:

The Darwin Effect

"The hardest person to be honest with on an everyday basis is ourself!"

~ Charles Weaver

The Herd Mentality was first put forward by 19th century social psychologists Gabriel Tarde and Gustave Le Bork. *The Herd Mentality* refers to the tendency to adopt the behavior and thinking of those around us and it is an ingrained part of our nature. In fact, there are certain situations where our social abilities can actually be a detriment to our individual success. This sense of belonging or going with the wave suppresses creativity, stops us from taking risks and experiencing failure, hurts our ability to achieve our goals, breeds an indifference towards understanding the world around us, and can lead us to become more conformist.

When we are with a group, whether it's a family, schoolmates, or work colleagues, we have a tendency to adopt the same behaviors and beliefs of others. This is clear when we see children copying the behavior of their parents and parents imitating their children. If someone in your circle has had success in something you want to do, it can be tempting to follow in their footsteps or adopt their practices without ever questioning the necessity or effectiveness of adopting such behavior in your own case. Our minds automatically compare ourselves with those around us because they are familiar and visible.

Psychologists call it the conformity bias or peer pressure. It's this tendency that leads us to wear the same brands, like the same activities, become friends with those who are similar to us, and even cultivate such tastes in the first place. In this way, we consciously or unconsciously copy the behavior of others and become more like them.

One day a lady was teaching her son and daughter how to bake a honey ham. The first step, she told the two, is to cut both ends of the ham off. She went on to explain every ingredient and every step thoroughly. Now she was about to place the ham in the oven, when her daughter asked why she cut the ends of the ham off. Frustrated by a seemingly dumb question her mom said, "YOU JUST DO! That is the way your grandmother taught me." This answer did not satisfy her curiosity so she went to her grandmother's house and asked her. She got the same answer in a sarcastic and frustrated tone, "YOU JUST DO! That is the way your great-grandmother taught me!" Still, her curiosity wasn't satisfied so she went to the nursing home and asked her great-grandmother why she cut the ends off the ham. She said with same sarcastic and frustrated tone, "SO IT WOULD FIT IN THE PAN!"

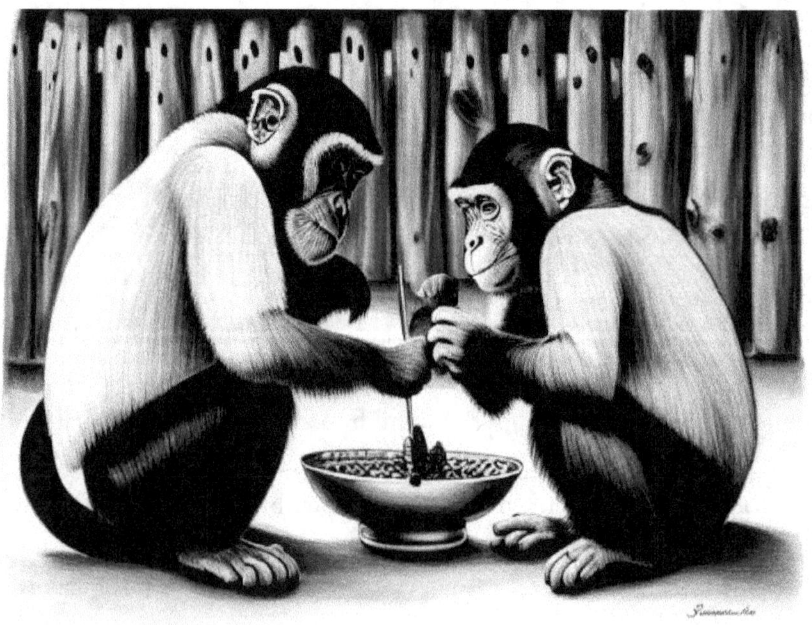

This next experiment should have never been allowed to take place and today it would not. It is the experiment called *5 Monkeys in a Cage*, which has been a controversial and oft-cited study in the field of psychology. Originally conducted by G.R. Stephenson in the 1960s, the experiment aimed to demonstrate the social transmission of learned behavior. While the experiment has been praised for its insights into the social dynamics of animal behavior, it has also been criticized for its ethical implications as it should. Yet, it gives us insights at the dangers and implications of not asking "why?"

The experiment involved placing five monkeys in a cage with a ladder leading up to a bunch of bananas. Whenever any of the monkeys tried to climb the ladder and reach for the bananas, they were sprayed with cold water. Over time, the monkeys learned to avoid the ladder and the bananas to prevent getting sprayed with cold water. One by one, the original monkeys were replaced with new monkeys. Every time the new monkey attempted to climb the ladder, the other monkeys would violently attack them. Over time, every time a monkey was replaced and the new monkey attempted to climb the ladder, the other monkeys would violently attack them, though none of the current monkeys had ever been sprayed by cold water. **NONE!**

The experiment has been widely cited as an example of social learning and the transmission of cultural knowledge within animal communities. However, it has also been criticized for its ethical implications, particularly with regard to animal welfare, and I totally agree. Some critics argue that the monkeys were subjected to unnecessary stress and discomfort and that the experiment raises serious questions about the humane treatment of animals in scientific research. I totally agree.

The power of suggestion is a phenomenon that has intrigued scientists and psychologists for decades. It is the ability of one person to influence the thoughts, feelings, and behaviors of another person through subtle cues and prompts. One of the most famous experiments on the power of suggestion was conducted by psychologist Solomon Asch in the 1950s. In this experiment, groups were shown a series of cards with lines of different lengths and were asked to identify the longest or shortest line. However, all but one of the participants were actually working for the experimenter and purposely gave wrong answers. As a result, the lone participant, who was not working for the experimenter, began to doubt their own judgments and conformed to the group's incorrect answer despite it obviously being wrong. This gives us yet further insight into the dangers of the herd mentality. It puts limits on us. Others can discourage our attempt at an endeavor in which they failed and quit.

Our Environment Shapes Us

The Darwin Effect is a term used to describe the idea that certain individuals or groups of people who are less adaptive or less fit will be weeded out by natural selection over time. This concept is based on the theories of Charles Darwin, who is famous for his work on evolution and the origin of species. The Darwin Effect is often used to explain why certain populations or species evolve and change over time while others become extinct or are unable to survive in changing environments. One example of the Darwin Effect can be seen in the case of the peppered moth in England. During the Industrial Revolution, pollution caused trees to darken, making it difficult for lighter-colored moths to blend in and avoid predators. As a result, darker-colored moths became more prevalent, as they were better able to survive in this new environment. This is an example of natural selection in action, as the traits that were most beneficial for survival became more common over time.

Another example of the Darwin Effect can be seen in the case of antibiotic resistance in bacteria. As antibiotics have become more widely used, bacteria have evolved to become resistant to them. This is because the bacteria that are able to survive exposure to antibiotics are the ones that will pass on their genes to the next generation. Over time, this can lead to the emergence of superbugs that are resistant to multiple types of antibiotics.

The point is that just because someone you know failed and quit doesn't mean you will fail or should quit. There are too many variables that you don't know about to base your decisions solely on the experiences of others. We should embrace being different and be cautious about any motivation that entices us to want to be like someone else.

Winning by Being Different

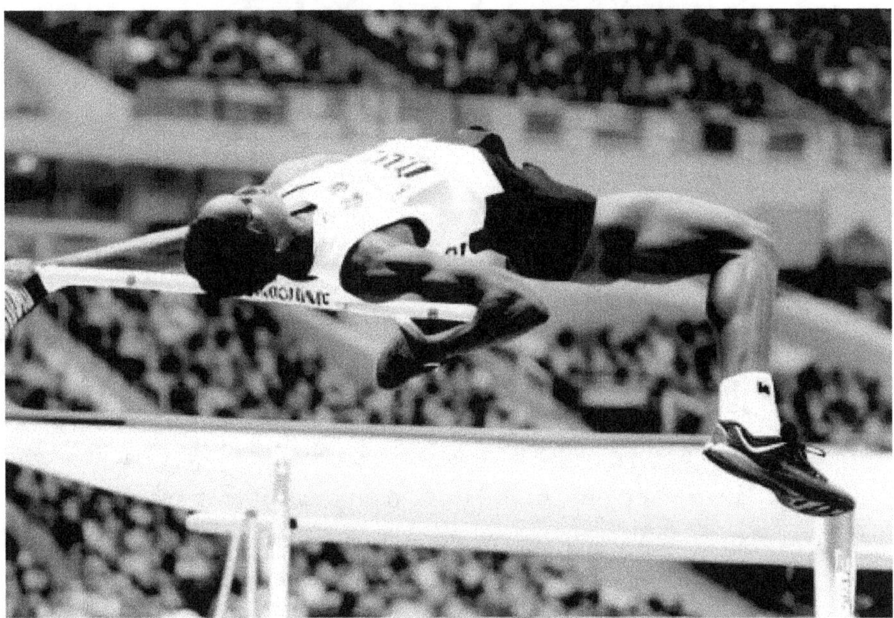

I believe when Einstein said that insanity is "doing the same thing over and over again and expecting different results," he was referring to the herd mentality. The term insanity can be replaced by conformity, uniformity, tradition, or copycat (Wilczek, 2015). Often, it's those who have accepted the status quo that are insane. After all, they are doing exactly what everyone else is doing. The herd mentality has a role in society because it helps us to get along and blend in easily with those around us, but if we allow ourselves to become too encumbered by conventionality, then we will never find true happiness and success. There are reasons why certain people have achieved more than others. As history shows us, it is those who dare to be different and embrace their own ambitions that makes the biggest mark on the world.

When it comes to success, people who have a clear plan and stick to it, will be more successful than those who think they are following a plan, but are actually just reacting to what others do. Dick Fosbury found a way to win though he was ridiculed for doing so along the way.

High jumping is an event in track and field athletics where athletes seek to jump over a horizontal bar resting upon two upright poles. The goal is to clear the bar without knocking it down using a technique that combines physical strength, agility, and coordination. This technique involves the approach, takeoff, and clearance.

Approach: Athletes use a run-up to generate speed and momentum towards the bar.

Takeoff: At the last moment, the athlete plants their foot and propels themselves upwards, converting horizontal velocity into vertical lift.

Clearance: Traditionally, high jumpers used either the scissors or straddle techniques to clear the bar.

Dick Fosbury decided to challenge the status quo and innovate the sport by introducing a unique style that defied convention. Coaches and teammates laughed at him because he didn't fall into their mold. The reason so many people quit, in my opinion, isn't because of adversity, but rather people trying to humiliate them. When you are being ridiculed you have to have massive amounts of intrinsic motivation to keep going. Dick Fosbury did and instead of taking a linear approach to jump, he arched his back and went over the bar backward, effectively going against the long-standing methods.

Fosbury stunned the world by winning the gold medal with a jump of 2.24 meters using his new technique in 1968 during the Olympic games in Mexico City. This marked the first time, what is now called the Fosbury Flop, was showcased on a global stage. Today, the Fosbury Flop is the gold standard for elite high jumpers all over the world.

Richard Branson's Virgin brand is synonymous with doing things differently, whether it's radical marketing strategies or simply creating a unique product that works better than its competitors. Richard Branson is a prominent example of how thinking differently can be successful. He built an empire from a student magazine and an airline with no airplanes! People see the success, but not the adversity he overcame. They thought he wasn't smart, and he left school at 15. He is brilliant, but his dyslexia made it extremely difficult for him to stand out academically in the traditional methods of the time. Albert Einstein wasn't just a brilliant scientist; he literally changed the world after dropping out of high school at 15 as well. Both kept going and over time their narrative changed.

Going against the grain can lead to criticism and even ridicule. In fact, the more someone goes against the grain, the more likely they are to come under scrutiny. People who rebel against the herd mentality stand out more than those who do the same things as everyone else. In some ways, it's the riskiest thing you can do. Most people won't take the time to understand what we're trying to accomplish or why we are trying to accomplish it. The reason is, God put that dream in our heart and not theirs. They can't get as excited as us and it is difficult for them to relate to our dream, much less understand why we keep fighting through adversity.

This brings us back to power vs force. The world will motivate us to be like them with force and if we don't embrace, build, and maintain our intrinsic motivation we are likely to conform to the *herd mentality.*

People who win by being different often come under criticism before those around them see the benefits of their approach. This is by design. We have to get push back and keep going to strengthen our intrinsic motivation. If everything worked out perfectly without a setback, we would not acquire the strength needed to sustain the success. When we reach a point where we feel stuck or beaten, that is when the real growth begins. I'm sure you know that feeling when you feel like all your hard work is unappreciated or even going to waste. In these situations, it's all too easy to give up on your dreams and let others have the final say in what you achieve.

It starts by acknowledging the narrative fallacy. Our brains love creating connections between random and unrelated things. We see connections where there are none, and we attribute meaning to randomness. We may start to assume that our business failed because we're not good enough or that our relationships fell apart because we're unlovable. These assumptions are part of the narrative fallacy, a cognitive bias that can hinder us from moving forward when faced with challenges (Penn, 2019).

Numerous psychological research papers point to the fact that we'll often link failure to some underlying internal persona. Of course, this is an illogical leap. It's easier to blame yourself than to think that random events are just that, random. We're also less willing to take risks when we fear failure. Research suggests that our fear of failure leads us to avoid failure at all costs, and in turn, we don't really live life at all. Instead, we conform.

This is what Theodore Roosevelt was alluding to when he delivered the speech entitled "Citizenship in the Republic" at the Sorbonne, in Paris, France, on April 23, 1910. The speech is largely known as "The Man in the Arena."

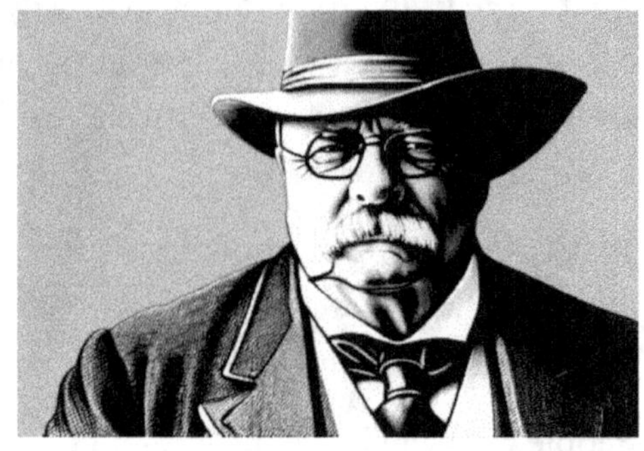

"It is not the critic who counts; not the man who points out how the strong man stumbles, or where the doer of deeds could have done them better. The credit belongs to the man who is actually in the arena, whose face is marred by dust and sweat and blood; who strives valiantly; who errs, who comes short again and again, because there is no effort without error and shortcoming; but who does actually strive to do the deeds; who knows great enthusiasms, the great devotions; who spends himself in a worthy cause; who at the best knows in the end the triumph of high achievement, and who at the worst, if he fails, at least fails while daring greatly, so that his place shall never be with those cold and timid souls who neither know victory nor defeat."

We become stronger and stronger when we realize that setbacks are necessary. What happens if we no longer fear them and rather see them as a chance to learn and grow? Back to our first example - Dick Fosbury. Although his unique style was ridiculed by his peers, he didn't let the criticism dampen his enthusiasm. He used it as fuel to keep moving forward, knowing that not everyone would understand his approach, including his own coach. He stayed true to himself, and in the end, he revolutionized the way people viewed high jumping forever.

Fortunately, we're in a position where we aren't restricted by the opinions of others. We all have the ability to carve our own path, and if we do it well, our actions can change the world for the better. The key is to focus on what we want to achieve and not on the adversity we face. We have the choice to confront challenges directly or to seek out obstacles and reasons for potential failure even before embarking on a new endeavor. Fears do not dictate our life when we have developed intrinsic motivation. We don't fail unless we quit. We are learning and getting stronger.

THOUGHTS

Chapter 7:

I Get What I Pay For Every Time

"According to all known laws of aviation, there is no way a bee should be able to fly. Its wings are too small to get its fat little body off the ground. The bee, of course, flies anyway, because bees don't care what humans think is impossible."

~ The Bee Movie (2007)

Decision Making

"Thinking, Fast and Slow" is a groundbreaking book written by Nobel laureate Daniel Kahneman. In this engaging and thought-provoking work, Kahneman explores the two systems of thinking that shape our decision-making processes. The book introduces two main concepts: System 1 and System 2. System 1 represents our fast, instinctive, and intuitive thinking, while System 2 represents our slow, deliberate, and logical thinking. Through various experiments and examples, Kahneman demonstrates how these two systems interact and influence our judgments and choices.

Kahneman delves into cognitive biases and heuristics that affect our decision-making, such as the availability heuristic and the anchoring effect we spoke of earlier. He also explores the role of emotions in decision-making and how they can lead to biases. One of the central themes of the book is the contrast between our irrational cognitive biases and the ideal of human rationality. Kahneman argues that our minds often rely on shortcuts and biases, leading to systematic errors. He presents numerous examples of these biases, including the impact of framing effects, loss aversion, and overconfidence.

Another key topic in the book is the concept of prospect theory, which challenges the traditional economic models of rational decision-making. Kahneman explains how individuals often make choices based on their perception of gains and losses rather than actual probabilities and outcomes. When we know what is challenging our ability to make the best decisions, we will be able to operate at our optimal cognitive level. Here are some of the main concepts he discusses.

The Halo Effect: Kahneman explains how our impressions of people and things can be influenced by an initial positive or negative attribute. This bias, known as the halo effect, can cloud our judgment and lead to inaccurate assessments.

The Power of Priming: The book explores the concept of priming, which refers to the subtle cues or stimuli that influence our subsequent thoughts and behaviors. Kahneman shares experiments that demonstrate how priming can impact our decision-making without our conscious awareness.

The Illusion of Understanding: Kahneman discusses how we often create coherent narratives in our mind even when faced with incomplete or ambiguous information. This illusion of understanding can lead to overconfidence and biases in our judgments.

The Role of Intuition: While intuition can be beneficial in certain situations, Kahneman warns that it can also lead to biases and errors. He emphasizes the importance of being aware of when to trust our intuition and when to engage in more deliberate thinking.

Loss Aversion: The book explores the concept of loss aversion, which suggests that people tend to strongly prefer avoiding losses over acquiring gains. This bias can influence our decision-making and make us more risk-averse.

The Availability Heuristic: Kahneman explains how the availability heuristic causes us to judge the frequency or likelihood of an event based on how easily examples or instances come to mind. This bias can lead to inaccurate assessments when we rely on easily accessible information.

Anchoring Effect: Kahneman describes how our judgments can be influenced by initial reference points, known as anchors. These anchors anchor our subsequent thoughts and evaluations, even when they are irrelevant or arbitrary.

These are just a few highlights from Daniel Kahneman's "Thinking, Fast and Slow." The book is rich in insights and examples, challenging our assumptions about human rationality and shedding light on the complex workings of our minds. Regardless, everything we get in life can be attributed to our focus, attitude, time and effort. Whether it be on making the most informed decisions or not. What we get in life is not limited to where we were born, the color of our skin or a perceived disability. If we use our FATE to learn how to optimize our decision-making skills, we will make better decisions. If we use our FATE on hate, we will become great at hating. If we use our FATE on our spiritual life we will have a great spiritual life. If we use our FATE on earning money, we will earn a lot of money.

F.A.T.E. is Purchasing Power

When we are positive, kind, and empathetic, we will attract people who are positive, kind, and empathetic. If you are happy and peaceful, then continue with the way you are spending your Focus, Attitude, Time, and Effort because that is as successful as you can become.

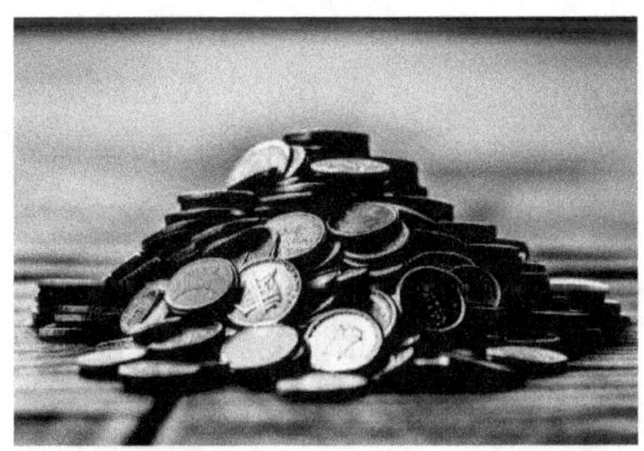

We have money that we spend as currency to trade for our basic necessities as well as items of luxury, vacations, etc. Few people ever realize we get that currency with our Focus, Attitude, Time, and Effort. While in college, I had a baseball coach who taught me how to set goals, which is why I respectfully disagree with how people set goals in business. He taught us that going to the Small College World Series was not the goal. Winning the conference was not the goal. The goal is to put in the effort to learn the proper fundamentals of fielding and hitting, as well as how to play the game properly, and practice so much that it becomes natural, which means performing without thought. The Navy Seals philosophy is we don't rise to the occasion. We fall to the level of preparation.

Let's take a professional sales career as an example. Upper management will give us production "goals." Production is a byproduct of Focus, Attitude, Time, and Effort. When we focus on the production goals, we tend to relax over time when we are close to that attainment. When the goal is Focus, Attitude, Time, and Effort, we set the curve. This means those who blow out their "number" aren't focusing on the number. Instead, they are focusing on what produces the number. Regarding sales, take the "number" and divide that by the number of presentations needed to accumulate that number of sales. It's not about pushing people or using manipulative practices. When we focus on the number, every NO stings a lot worse than focusing on the activity that achieves the "number." The number is a byproduct of our plan. When we get punched in the mouth, we are more likely to keep moving forward instead of looking for another job. While playing baseball, if we made an error, we were not allowed to get down, frustrated, or angry at ourselves or a teammate, because we knew how to fix it, and the windshield was bigger than the rearview mirror on purpose. We never let one loss beat us twice.

Everything we have in life is purchased with our Focus, Attitude, Time, and Effort, and these are finite. Our marriage, relationships, ability to be a high achiever and our income are all purchased with our F.A.T.E. We purchase everything we have, even our relationship with God. Our true currency is not money. Instead, it is our Focus, Attitude, Time, and Effort.

Jim Kwik's childhood was marked by his struggles with learning disabilities, including dyslexia and ADHD. Born in the late 1970s in San Bernardino, California, Jim Kwik faced many challenges in his early years. However, his experiences with these challenges would eventually lead him to his life's work - helping others unlock the full potential of their brains. As a child, Jim Kwik struggled to read and write. He often had trouble focusing and retaining information, which made it difficult for him to keep up with his classmates. His teachers and parents saw him as a slow learner, and he was often criticized for his academic performance. Jim Kwik's struggles with learning disabilities caused him a great deal of frustration and shame.

However, it was a traumatic event that ultimately led Jim Kwik to discover his passion for accelerated learning. One day, when he was in the fourth grade, Jim Kwik fell off his bike and suffered a serious head injury. After the accident, he experienced memory loss and had trouble remembering basic information like his phone number and address. This experience left a lasting impression on Jim Kwik and sparked his interest in the power of the brain. Jim Kwik was determined to overcome his learning disabilities and improve his brain performance. He began to study different learning techniques, including speed reading and memory improvement. By the time he was in high school, he had become an expert in these areas and began to tutor his classmates. His passion for learning led him to pursue a degree in neuroscience and psychology at the University of California, Los Angeles (UCLA). While at UCLA, he began to develop his own unique approach to learning, which he later called the Kwik Learning Method.

Jim Kwik's childhood experiences with learning disabilities have played a significant role in shaping his career. He has become a leading expert in the field of accelerated learning, memory improvement, and brain performance and has helped thousands of people around the world overcome their own learning challenges. In his latest book, "Limitless: Upgrade Your Brain, Learn Anything Faster, and Unlock Your Exceptional Life," Jim Kwik shares his personal story of how he overcame his learning disabilities and dyslexia to become a successful entrepreneur and world-renowned speaker. He encourages readers to embrace their own limitations and use them as a catalyst for growth and self-improvement.

Do you think he would have ever achieved this level of success if he wasn't forced to overcome his learning disabilities? Maybe. Don't get me wrong. I think it was the traumatic experience that ultimately caused him to become so focused on learning, but I doubt that he would have been the same person if he wasn't forced to develop those skills. We all go through tough times, and most of the time, it's life that forces us to become stronger and improve our plan, and move forward.

Adversity means different things to different people. To me, it's a seed, and peace is its fruit. To others, it might be a sign that they should quit their job and start their own business, or it might be something that forces them to rethink their life goals. It's all about perspective. The adversity we experience in life will dictate how we react and change our lives for the better. Adversity is a good thing.

Jim Kwik has learned a lot from his childhood struggles with learning disabilities. He takes those experiences and turns them into fuel, fueling his motivation and passion for growing greater success in his life, professionally and personally. If we have nothing to look forward to, we have no reason to look forward, and adversity will be our demise. If we feel like it's a dog-eat-dog world and we are wearing milk bone underwear, then we have to find something to look forward to, or we will spend all of our time looking backward.

If we choose to see the challenge in front of us as fuel and we put in the effort to overcome it, we will reap the rewards. It's all about how we frame things, and I saw it firsthand in college. My roommate had gained a lot of weight. People would pick on him, saying he had *"done lap disease because the top of his jeans done lapped over his belt."*

It was true. Even after they came out of the washer and dryer, they had a permanent crease. That was his tipping point. One day, I saw a brand-new pair of running shoes beside his bed. I'm not proud of this, but I laughed because I sincerely thought that someone had left them in our room. He wasn't amused, but chose to react in a rather interesting way. He taught me a lifelong lesson. I asked, "Are you running miles now?" He said, "Not now, but I don't have to be able to run a mile today to be able to run a mile. MY GOAL is to run to one more mailbox every day." Birch Gentry is now a very successful pharmacist in Nashville, Tennessee. Later, I learned a similar quote from Dr. MLK. "You don't have to see the top of the stairs to get there. Just keep taking the next step." There must be a tipping point for the attitude change. Then, bite- sized chunks for an extended period of time. The point is you don't stop trying because you couldn't learn the way you were being taught. Find another teacher! Find someone who has overcome what you are dealing with. 2B1Ask1

While vacationing in The Dominican Republic, I realized those working the landscape did not have a very good attitude. Not that they were offensive, but they were not in a good mood. I mentioned to our concierge, Anibal, how working the gardens must be very hard work because of the attitudes I observed. He told me that is where we all start. I was confused. He explained that everyone started cleaning rooms and cleaning the grounds. Only those with the best attitudes get to move up. Genius. An attitude factory. The staff, not the management, lives by a saying.

"Don't wait for life to stop being hard to start being happy."

The Secret by Rhonda Byrne has gone beyond just being a book. It has become a worldwide phenomenon, leading to the creation of a documentary film, audio recordings, and even a follow-up book titled "The Power," which further explores the principles of the law of attraction. The Secret documentary, released in 2000, features interviews with various authors, philosophers, and motivational speakers who share their insights on attraction. It provides a visual representation of the concepts discussed in the book and includes real-life individuals who have applied these teachings to achieve extraordinary success and happiness.

The popularity of The Secret has led to the formation of numerous online communities and social media groups dedicated to discussing and practicing the principles taught in the book. These platforms serve as a support system where individuals can share their experiences, seek guidance, and motivate one another to stay committed to their goals.

Furthermore, The Secret has inspired countless other self-help authors, speakers, and coaches to incorporate the principles of the law of attraction into their work. Numerous seminars and retreats have been organized worldwide, providing individuals with the opportunity to deepen their understanding of the law of attraction and learn practical techniques to manifest their desires. The Secret has sparked important conversations and inspired individuals around the world to take back control of their lives and pursue their dreams.

When we dare to be different and/or dare to be great we have to "learn outside of the box." Everyone else is learning at work and during school. What separates us from *the herd* are the books we read, the podcasts we listen to and our desire to learn outside of work and/or school. It's just a little "extra" that turns ordinary, into extraordinary.

THOUGHTS

Chapter 8:

Mental Health And Conflicts

"Mental health is not a destination, but a process. It's about how you drive, not where you are going."

~ Noam Shpancer

Mental health is a crucial aspect of overall well-being, yet it is often overlooked and/or marginalized. Every person on the planet has bouts where their mental health is challenged and even situations where it is damaged. We are not alone, so instead of acting like it doesn't exist, let's talk about it. Former heavyweight boxing champion Mike Tyson said it like this, "Everyone has a plan until they get punched in the mouth." Since we know when we make a plan, we are going to get punched in the mouth, why don't we make a plan for getting back up?

Then there are those times when we get hit in the mouth and don't see it coming. When my mom passed, I was in a dark place. I've had my share of trauma in life, but nothing like this because she was always there during those times. I had no problem going to talk to someone or a therapist, but when I went to look, it was very difficult to find someone with an immediate opening and for a fee I felt was reasonable. Humans are not designed to be alone, and when we are in dark times, we feel alone because few of us have social groups that contain trained professionals to whom we can reach out for help. However, I told my family practice doctor, and he led me to a telehealth therapist.

That is when I met Carlos Castanada in Austin, Texas. I was able to schedule several appointments through video chat and it was super convenient and affordable. He didn't just listen to me and give me advice. He explained how the brain deals with traumatic events and gave me exercises to do for acute episodes, as well as exercises for my chronic episodes. It was literally a life-changing experience. No longer did I feel weak or less than those around me; I felt empowered. I no longer felt alone, especially realizing that everyone has acute episodes and most people have chronic episodes of poor mental health.

The World Health Organization defines mental health as a state of well-being in which the individual realizes his or her own abilities, can cope with the normal stresses of life, can work productively and fruitfully, and is able to make a contribution to his or her community. Fortunately, there are numerous evidence-based strategies that promote mental well-being and reduce the impact of mental health issues.

Self-care involves deliberately engaging in activities that promote physical, mental, and emotional well-being. This involves light exercise, proper nutrition, adequate sleep, mindfulness practices, and leisure activities. When I say exercise, I do not mean running a marathon. We can go for a walk. Research has consistently shown that self-care activities are essential to improving mental health, reducing stress levels (Chiesa & Serretti, 2018), and increasing resilience (Harris et al., 2018).

Building and maintaining strong connections is crucial for mental health. Friends or support groups provide emotional support, a sense of belonging, and a space to share experiences and challenges. Social support has been linked to reduced mental health episodes (Lunstad et al., 2010) and improved recovery from existing mental health conditions (Cohen, 2004). It is essential to prioritize meaningful relationships and seek support when needed, and if you can't figure out how to belong to a social group, go volunteer for a couple of hours a month.

Mind and meditation practices involve focusing one's attention on the present moment and a non-judgmental awareness of thoughts and feelings. These have been found to reduce symptoms of anxiety and depression while improving overall mental well-being (Khourly et al., 2013).

Incorporating mindfulness into daily life through meditation, breathing, or mindful walks can lead to significant improvements in mental health. You can get started from your living room couch. Go to YouTube and search. You will find more how-to videos than you can watch in a lifetime.

Regular physical activity has numerous mental health benefits. We release endorphins and feel-good hormones, improve mood, and reduce symptoms of depression and anxiety (Stanton & Reaburn, 2014). It also promotes better sleep, increases self-esteem, and enhances cognitive function (Angevaren et al., 2008). Finding enjoyable activities such as walking, dancing, or team sports can make physical activity more sustainable. If you're not athletic, give pickle ball a chance.

Grateful people become successful, successful people don't become grateful. Practicing gratitude involves intentionally focusing on the positive aspects of life and acknowledging the things for which one is grateful. Research has shown that gratitude interventions can improve mental health, including well-being, satisfaction with life, and positive emotions (Wood et al., 2010). A simple yet effective way to express gratitude is by keeping a gratitude journal on three things for which one is grateful. Every day you write it down. How do you know 100% if it works? Don't tell anyone. Start and wait for people to start commenting on how there is something different about you, but they can't tell what. BOOM!

Finding a balance between work and personal life for mental well- being isn't a choice. It's essential. Overworking and neglecting personal needs will lead to burnout, stress, and a decline in mental health. Engaging in activities outside of work will help you perform better at work, decrease stress, and increase overall well-being.

Excessive screen time and digital overload have been associated with adverse mental health effects, such as decreased well-being and increased symptoms of depression and anxiety. Setting time limits for screen usage, taking regular breaks, and participating in offline activities will help reduce the negative impact of technology on mental health overall. This is another reason volunteering is so nutritious.

If struggling with mental health issues, seeking professional help is crucial.

Mental health professionals, such as psychologists, counselors, or psychiatrists, can provide support, therapy, and, if necessary, medication. Early intervention can prevent the worsening of mental health conditions and begin recovery. Consulting with a qualified professional ensures evidence-based interventions to your individual needs.

Improving mental health requires a holistic approach that encompasses various aspects of life. Prioritizing self-care, seeking social support, practicing mindfulness, engaging in physical activity, and establishing work-life balance are a few strategies that can significantly enhance mental well-being. It is essential to remember that everyone's journey to mental health is unique, and what works for one person may not work for another. Experimentation and ongoing self-reflection are key to discovering the most effective strategies for individual mental health improvement.

A healthy diet plays a vital role in mental health. Consuming nutrient- rich foods, such as fruits, vegetables, grains, lean proteins, and healthy fats, can support brain function and overall well-being. Research suggests that certain nutrients, such as omega-3 fatty acids, are particularly beneficial for mental health. We are all addicted to sugar before we can walk, but avoiding excessive sugar, processed foods, and alcohol can also contribute to better mental health. Incorporating relaxation techniques into daily life can help reduce stress and anxiety and promote mental well-being. Techniques like deep breathing exercises, progressive muscle relaxation, guided imagery, and yoga have been shown to have a positive impact on mental health. Again, YouTube is free, anonymous, and at your fingertips. Regular practice of these techniques can induce a state of calmness and improve sleep quality. Lack of sleep quality has been linked to a decrease in mental health wellbeing, including depression disorders (Pillai et al., 2018). Establishing a consistent sleep routine, creating a sleep-conducive environment, and practicing relaxation techniques at bedtime can promote better sleep, hygiene, and overall mental well-being.

Chronic stress will negatively impact our physical health. We can use mental stress management techniques, such as time management, setting boundaries, practicing mindfulness, and engaging in relaxation exercises. Yet, these techniques will alleviate acute stress, but they will never be enough for the long-term improvement of chronic stress.

Improving mental health for long-term well-being involves care, seeking social support, practicing mindfulness, engaging in physical activity, maintaining a healthy work-life balance, and incorporating other strategies like proper nutrition and relaxation techniques. It is important to remember that each person's journey toward mental health may vary, and seeking professional help when needed is not only okay, but it should be planned. By implementing these evidence- based strategies, we can take significant steps toward improving our mental health and overall quality of life.

"Hope and Help for Your Nerves" by Dr. Claire Weekes is a groundbreaking book that offers valuable strategies for overcoming anxiety and its debilitating effects. Weekes, a renowned Australian doctor and specialist in anxiety disorders, provides a comprehensive guide to understanding anxiety in a compassionate and accessible manner. The book begins by acknowledging the pervasive nature of anxiety and its impact on one's physical, emotional, and psychological well- being. Weekes highlights that anxiety is a common human experience and assures readers that they are not alone in their struggle. By normalizing anxiety as a natural response to stress and uncertainty, she helps alleviate the shame and stigma often associated with mental health. Dr. Weekes has an uncanny ability to explain complex concepts in a relatable manner. She breaks down the science behind anxiety, explaining the physiological changes that occur in the body during anxious episodes. Through her clear explanations, readers gain a deeper understanding of the mechanisms underlying their anxiety, empowering them to take control of their own healing process.

Weekes emphasizes the importance of acceptance as a crucial step towards recovery. She encourages readers to embrace their anxiety rather than resist it. By accepting their anxiety, individuals can free themselves from the cycle of fear and avoidance that often perpetuates the condition. This approach aligns with the principles of mindfulness and self-compassion, which have been shown to be effective in managing anxiety.

Furthermore, the book provides numerous practical strategies for coping with anxiety. Weekes outlines various relaxation techniques, breathing exercises, and progressive muscle relaxation that enable us to calm our bodies and minds during anxious moments. She also offers guidance on how to identify negative thought patterns and replace them with more positive and realistic beliefs.

Weekes' approach is holistic, addressing the physical, cognitive, and emotional aspects of anxiety. She recognizes the interconnectedness of these dimensions and emphasizes the need for a comprehensive approach to healing. Overall, Hope and Help for Your Anxiety stands as a timeless resource for us all during our struggles. Weekes' compassionate and knowledgeable approach, combined with practical strategies and relatable examples, makes this book an invaluable tool for those seeking to overcome and reclaim their lives.

The smarter we are, the harder it is to find peace because we can see more injustices to us and others. Yet, when we learn, adapt, and adjust, we can use our mental health to improve everything about our lives. I once heard someone say, "To be a leader, you have to be a reader." They were talking about leading others at work, but I think reading and learning are even more important for us to lead ourselves throughout the day.

There are businesses that only interview candidates who have volunteer experience on their resume, and there is a reason. Susan Albers, PsyD, a psychologist from the esteemed Cleveland Clinic, who studied the benefits of volunteering, has found that volunteering has long been recognized as a worthwhile and enriching activity that benefits both individuals and communities, offering a profound impact on our mental and emotional well-being. Volunteering offers a unique opportunity to society, while nurturing our own mental health.

Albers says that engaging in acts of kindness and altruism activates the pleasure centers in the brain, leading to a release of feel-good hormones like dopamine and oxytocin. These neurochemicals not only enhance our mood, but also reduce stress and anxiety levels.

Dr. Albers cites several studies demonstrating that individuals who regularly volunteer are less likely to experience chronic depression, anxiety, and loneliness. By connecting with others and engaging in meaningful activities, volunteers cultivate a sense of purpose and belonging, which are key factors in maintaining good mental health. One of the most significant benefits of volunteering, as highlighted by Dr. Albers, is its potential to forge strong social connections and camaraderie in the community.

"The strongest people are not those who show strength in front of us but those who win battles we know nothing about."

Jonathan Harnisch

Through volunteering, individuals have the opportunity to meet like-minded people who share similar interests. This shared sense of purpose and collaboration not only creates a supportive network, but also helps combat feelings of isolation and loneliness. Engaging in volunteer work often involves learning new skills or honing existing ones, which have a positive impact on our growth. Dr. Albers emphasizes how the acquisition of new knowledge and abilities through volunteering can boost self-confidence and self-esteem.

Volunteer opportunities offer a safe and supportive environment to step out of our comfort zone, create healthy challenges, and the opportunity to learn from others. As a result, volunteers often develop a greater sense of self-efficacy and belief in their abilities, which positively impact other areas of life as well. Volunteering exposes us to diverse cultures, perspectives, and life experiences that we may not encounter in our everyday lives. Dr. Albers asserts that this exposure fosters empathy, compassion, and gratitude. When we witness the struggles and triumphs of others, we gain a broader perspective on our own and develop a deeper appreciation for our lives. These new perspectives lead to increased positivity, resilience, and a greater sense of gratitude. Volunteermatch.org is a great place to get started.

Nothing can challenge mental health like a conflict at work and/or at home, but they can also be beneficial. Conflict is an inevitable part of life. It can arise from differences in opinions, values, interests, and goals between individuals or groups who have **ELEPHANT HEAD**. If these conflicts are not managed properly, they can lead to negative consequences such as damaged relationships, decreased productivity, and increased stress levels. Therefore, it is essential to develop effective conflict resolution strategies to address and resolve conflicts in a constructive manner. Before delving into conflict resolution strategies, it is crucial to understand the nature of conflicts. According to Difficult Conversations: *"How to Discuss What Matters Most,"* by Douglas Stone, Bruce Patton, Sheila Heen and Roger Fisher, Conflicts can be categorized into three main types:

Task conflicts: These conflicts arise from differences in opinions about work-related tasks such as goals, processes, or methods. Task conflicts can actually be beneficial as they encourage critical thinking and can lead to innovative solutions.

Relationship conflicts: Relationship conflicts occur when there are issues, such as personality clashes or personal animosity, between groups. These conflicts can be detrimental to productivity and teamwork.

Process conflicts: Process conflicts involve disagreements about how tasks or decisions should be accomplished. They often arise from differences in communication styles, decision- making, or resource allocation. Conflict resolution is an essential skill in our personal and professional lives, and there are several reasons for effective conflict resolution.

Resolving conflicts in a constructive manner can lead to stronger and healthier relationships. By addressing underlying issues and finding common ground, conflicts can be transformed into opportunities for growth and understanding. Also, conflict resolution encourages open and honest communication. It provides a platform for individuals to express their concerns and perspectives, fostering a better understanding of each other's viewpoints.

When conflicts are effectively resolved, it reduces tension and fosters a more collaborative work environment. This, in turn, enhances productivity and creativity within teams and organizations. Conflict resolution allows for a thorough exploration of different perspectives and a consideration of various options. This leads to more informed decision-making and better outcomes. Always remember, when emotions are high logic is low. Tone of voice and listening to understand vs waiting to respond are the most important elements to conflict resolution. There are several conflict resolution strategies that can be employed to effectively manage and resolve conflicts:

1. Creative Problem Solving

Creative problem-solving involves working together to find a mutually acceptable solution. This strategy requires active listening, empathy, and a focus on understanding each other's needs and interests. By exploring and integrating different perspectives, individuals can come up with solutions that satisfy everyone involved. The challenge here is listening to understand versus waiting to respond.

Example: Imagine two colleagues have differing opinions on the implementation of a new marketing strategy. Instead of arguing or dismissing each other's ideas, they engage in collaborative problem-solving. They actively listen to each other's perspectives, understand each other's concerns, and collaborate to find a solution that incorporates the best aspects of their ideas.

2. Compromise

Compromise involves finding a middle ground between positions. It requires a willingness to give up some of one's own preferences in order to reach an agreement. Compromise can be a useful strategy when the stakes are not high, and both parties are to make concessions. The challenge here is listening to understand versus waiting to respond. If you are unaware that you are in a state of waiting to respond and/or using a high tone of voice, you might unknowingly play a significant role in fueling the conflict, my friend.

Example: In a business negotiation, two parties have different expectations regarding the price of a product. After discussing their concerns and exploring various options, they reach a compromise by settling on a price that is acceptable to both parties.

3. Assertiveness and Active Listening

Assertiveness and active listening are crucial skills in conflict resolution.

Assertiveness involves expressing one's needs, thoughts, and concerns clearly and respectfully. Active listening, on the other hand, involves paying full attention to the speaker, paraphrasing, and summarizing their message to ensure understanding. The challenge here is listening to understand versus waiting to respond. If you are unaware that you are in a state of waiting to respond and/or using a high tone of voice, you might unknowingly play a significant role in fueling the conflict, my friend.

Example: In a team meeting, two team members' ideas regarding the allocation of resources are at odds with one another. Instead of talking over each other or disregarding each other's opinions, they practice assertiveness and active listening. They take turns expressing their viewpoints, ensuring that each person feels heard and understood.

4. Mediation

Mediation involves the presence of a neutral third party to help facilitate communication and negotiation between conflicting parties. The mediator does not impose decisions, but helps individuals or groups find common ground and reach a mutually satisfactory resolution. The challenge here is listening to understand versus waiting to respond. If you are unaware that you are in a state of waiting to respond and/or using a high tone of voice, you might unknowingly play a significant role in fueling the conflict, my friend.

Example: In a family conflict, two siblings are constantly arguing about household chores. Their parents intervene and act as mediators, facilitating a calm and respectful discussion between the siblings. The parents help them identify their underlying concerns and guide them toward finding a solution that works for both of them.

5. Avoidance and Accommodation

While not always the most effective, avoidance and accommodation can be useful in certain situations. Avoidance involves temporarily putting the conflict aside to allow emotions to cool down, while accommodation involves giving in to the other party's demands in order to maintain harmony. However, it is important to note that avoiding or accommodating conflicts for an extended period can lead to unresolved issues and resentment. The challenge here is listening to understand versus waiting to respond. If you are unaware that you are in a state of waiting to respond and/or using a high tone of voice, you might unknowingly play a significant role in fueling the conflict, my friend.

Example: In a workplace, two employees have a conflict over how to finish a project. As a temporary measure, they decide to put the discussion on hold and focus on other tasks to give them time to reflect on their own perspectives and emotions with a calmer mindset before revisiting the conflict.

Conflict resolution is a vital skill in both our personal and professional lives. By understanding the nature of conflicts and employing effective conflict resolution strategies, we can transform conflicts into opportunities for growth, improved relationships, and enhanced productivity. Whether through collaborative problem-solving, compromise, assertiveness, active listening, mediation, or avoidance and accommodation, conflicts can be resolved in a constructive manner. Ultimately, the goal of conflict resolution is to find mutually acceptable solutions that address the underlying issues and foster understanding and cooperation. Again, the two most important keys are listening to understand and speaking in a low tone of voice.

The secret is understanding our brain's instinct to respond to the behavior of others. When we have an unexpected encounter with another person, our brain instinctively wants to respond in a similar manner. The concept of reciprocity, a fundamental principle in social psychology, postulates that individuals tend to reciprocate gestures received from others in social interactions. Simply put, if someone does us a favor, we are inclined to do something in return for them. If someone is mad, we are inclined to become angry. If someone raises their voice, we are inclined to raise our voice. Understanding this basic fundamental principle in social psychology is paramount in successful conflict resolution. For example, our brain wants to respond in kind with a positive gesture or to make an additional purchase. Even if you are extremely angry when someone is nice to you, your brain wants to respond accordingly with a nice gesture. The problem is, if someone acts aggressively toward us, our brain wants to reciprocate with aggressive behavior toward them. Understanding what the brain wants and that reciprocating will implore the situation to escalate, possibly out of control, is the emotional intelligence needed for successful conflict resolution.

In his book " Split the Difference: Negotiating As If Your Life Depended On It," FBI hostage negotiator Chris Voss presents a revolutionary approach to negotiation. Drawing on his extensive experience in high-stakes negotiations, he offers practical strategies and techniques that can be applied not only in life-threatening situations, but also in everyday life. Voss starts by highlighting the importance of emotional intelligence in negotiations. According to him, emotions play a significant role in decision-making, and understanding how to influence them is crucial for successful negotiations. He introduces the concept of "tactical empathy," which involves understanding the emotions and perspectives of the other party. By practicing active listening and displaying genuine empathy, negotiators can build trust and establish rapport.

One of the key principles Voss emphasizes is the importance of "anchoring." Anchoring is the act of establishing a starting point for negotiations, often through making an extreme offer or asking for an unexpected task. This technique sets the tone and influences the perception of the negotiation's value. Voss advises negotiators to anchor aggressively, but always be prepared to adjust their position as the negotiation progresses. Voss also introduces the concept of "labeling," which involves verbalizing the emotions and fears of the other party. I call this the pink elephant in the room. Just call it out because by acknowledging and labeling these emotions, negotiators can create a sense of understanding and validation.

Another technique highlighted in the book is the use of calibrated questions. These questions, which are open-ended and begin with "how" or "what," force the other party to reflect and share valuable information. This also helps build rapport and keep the negotiation focused on the other party's perspective, increasing the chances of reaching a mutually beneficial agreement.

Voss also emphasizes the importance of "mirroring" as a powerful tool in negotiation. Mirroring involves repeating the last few words or paraphrasing the other party's statement. This technique not only shows that you are actively listening, but can also encourage the other party to expand on their thoughts and provide more information.

Additionally, Voss discusses the relevance of "negotiation as a process" rather than focusing on the outcome, which encourages negotiators to focus on the relationship and dynamics rather than solely on demands and concessions. By creating an environment and problem-solving, negotiators can increase the likelihood of reaching a win-win outcome. Emotional intelligence is crucial in negotiations because understanding and influencing the emotions of the other party is essential for success. By practicing active listening, negotiators can establish rapport and build trust. The techniques and strategies presented in "Never Split the Difference" can be applied in various real-world scenarios, such as:

Business Negotiations: Whether it's negotiating a deal, salary, or contract terms, the principles outlined in the book can help you navigate outcomes in business negotiations.

Conflict Resolution: The techniques presented in the book can be used to resolve conflicts and disagreements effectively, whether in personal relationships or professional settings.

Sales and Marketing: Understanding the emotions and perspectives of customers can help improve sales and marketing strategies. The information in the book can be applied to influence buying decisions and build stronger customer relationships.

Understanding the tendencies of our subconscious mind and how to manipulate them enriches our lives on several fronts. Yes, we build stronger relationships in both our personal and professional lives, but it also opens up a new frontier of what we are actually capable of, letting us dream bigger dreams and set bigger goals. More than anything, it lets us know we are okay. Even if we were born into a challenging environment or we struggled with anxiety or experienced trauma, we not only have a chance, we have a future!!

THOUGHTS

References

Grosso, G., Pajak, A., Marventano, S. et al. (2014). Role of omega-3 fatty acids in the treatment of depressive disorders: a comprehensive meta-analysis of randomized clinical trials. PLoS ONE, 9(5), e96905.

Hoge, E. A., Bui, E., Marques, L. et al. (2013). Randomized Controlled Trial of Mindfulness Meditation for Generalized Anxiety Disorder: Effects on Anxiety and Stress Reactivity. Journal of Consulting and Clinical Psychology, 82(6), 1180–1188.

Khoury, B., Lecomte, T., Fortin, G. et al. (2013). Mindfulness-based therapy: a comprehensive meta-analysis. Clinical Psychology Review, 33(6), 763–771.

Lopresti, A. L., Hood, S. D., & Drummond, P. D. (2013). A review of lifestyle factors that contribute to important pathways associated with major depression: diet, sleep, and exercise. Journal of Affective Disorders, 148(1), 12–27.

Matsuoka, Y. J., Sawada, N., Mimura, M. et al. (2018). Dietary intake of fish or n-3 polyunsaturated fatty acids and depressive symptoms: A systematic review and dose- response meta-analysis of observational studies. Journal of Affective Disorders, 235, 11–16.

Schuch, F. B., Vancampfort, D., Rosenbaum, S. et al. (2016). Exercise for depression in older adults: a meta-analysis of randomized controlled trials adjusting for publication bias. Brazilian Journal of Psychiatry, 38(3), 247–254.

Skarupski, K. A., Tangney, C., Li, H. et al. (2010). Longitudinal association of vitamin B-6, folate, and vitamin B-12 with depressive symptoms among older adults over time. American Journal of Clinical Nutrition, 92(2), 330–335.

Coussens, L. M., & Werb, Z. (2002). Inflammation and cancer. Nature, 420(6917), 860–867.

Lustig, R. H., Schmidt, L. A., & Brindis, C. D. (2012). Public health: The toxic truth about sugar. Nature, 482(7383), 27–29.

Malik, V. S., Popkin, B. M., Bray, G. A., Després, J.-P., Willett, W. C., & Hu, F. B. (2010). Sugar-sweetened beverages and risk of metabolic syndrome and type 2 diabetes: A meta-analysis. Diabetes Care, 33(11), 2477–2483.

Messier, C. (2010). Impact of impaired glucose tolerance and type 2 diabetes on cognitive aging. Neurobiology of Aging, 31(2), 175–183.

Moynihan, P., & Petersen, P. E. (2018). Diet, nutrition, and the prevention of dental diseases. Public Health Nutrition, 7(1a), 201–226.

Popkin, B. M., Hawkes, C., & Sweeting, A. N. (2012). Current

Hawkins, D. R. (2014). Power vs. Force: The Hidden Determinants of Human Behavior. Hay House, Inc.

Hayes, C., Strosahl, K., & Wilson, K. (2012). Acceptance and Commitment Therapy, Second Edition: The Process and Practice of Mindful Change. Guilford Press.

McLeod, S. A. (2013). Maslow's Hierarchy of Needs. Simply Psychology. Grenville-Cleave, L. (2020). The Science of Happiness. Positive Psychology.

Vanderbilt, T. (2011). The Power of Habit: Why We Do What We Do in Life and Business. Random House.

Kirsch, I. (1997). Specifying nonspecifics: Psychological mechanisms of placebo effects. In The science of the placebo: Toward an interdisciplinary research agenda (pp. 164-175). London: BMJ Books.

Colloca, L., & Benedetti, F. (2005). Placebos and painkillers: is mind as real as matter? Nature Reviews Neuroscience, 6(7), 545-552.

Finniss, D. G., Kaptchuk, T. J., Miller, F., & Benedetti, F. (2010)

"Roger Bannister, First Athlete to Run a Mile in Under Four Minutes, Dies at 88", The NewYork Times, 4 March 2018, https://www.nytimes.com/2018/03/04/obituaries/roger-bannister-dead.html.

"Roger Bannister: The man who broke the 4-minute mile", BBC Sport, 5 May 2004, https://www.bbc.com/sport/athletics/27118045

"Roger Bannister's four-minute mile: The impossible feat," CNN, 4 May 2014, https://edition.cnn.com/2014/05/06/sport/athlete-roger-bannister-four-minute-mile- anniversary-spt-intl/index.html

Ericsson, K. A., Krampe, R. T., & Tesch-Römer, C. (1993). The role of deliberate practice in the acquisition of expert performance. Psychological Review, 100(3), 363–

406. https://doi.org/10.1037/0033-295X.100.3.363 Gladwell, M. (2008). Outliers. Little, Brown and Company.

Asch, S. E. (1951). Effects of group pressure upon the modification and distortion of judgments. In H. Guetzkow (Ed.), Groups, leadership and men: Research in human relations (pp. 177-190). Carnegie Press.

Cialdini, R. B. (2007). Influence: The psychology of persuasion. HarperCollins. Levine, J. M., & Moreland, R. L. (2014). Small groups. Routledge.

Stephenson, G.R. (1967). "Cultural acquisition of a specific learned response among rhesus monkeys." In: Starek, D., Schneider, R., and Kuhn, H. J. (eds.), Progress in Primatology (pp. 279-288). Stuttgart: Fischer Verlag.

Morgan, C.L. (2005). "Monkey see, monkey avoid: The social transmission of learned behavior in primates." In: Trends in Cognitive Sciences 9.3 (pp. 122-124).

Mayo Clinic Staff. (2019). Cortisol level test. Mayo Clinic. https://www.mayoclinic.org/tests-procedures/cortisol-levels/about/pac-20384775

Chrousos, G. P. (2009). Stress and disorders of the stress system. Nature Reviews Endocrinology, 5(7), 374-381.

https://www.ncbi.nlm.nih.gov/pmc/articles/PMC2929498/

McEwen, B. S. (2007). Physiology and neurobiology of stress and adaptation: Central role of the brain. Physiological

Reviews, 87(3), 873-904. https://www.ncbi.nlm.nih.gov/pmc/articles/PMC2684060/

Cohen, S., Janicki-Deverts, D., & Miller, G. E. (2007). Psychological stress and disease. JAMA, 298(14), 1685-1687. https://jamanetwork.com/journals/jama/fullarticle

American Psychological Association. (2018). Understanding and Managing Anxiety. https://www.apa.org/topics/anxiety

American Psychological Association. (2021). The Fight or Flight Response. https://www.apa.org/topics/fight-or-flight

Cannon, W. B. (1929). Bodily changes in pain, hunger, fear, and rage: An account of recent researches into the function of emotional excitement. Appleton-Century.

Hofmann, S. G. (2007). Cognitive factors that maintain social anxiety disorder: A comprehensive model and its treatment implications. Cognitive Behaviour Therapy, 36(4), 193-209.

LeDoux, J. (2015). Anxious: Using the brain to understand and treat fear and anxiety. Penguin.

Henshaw, J. M., & Freedman-Doan, C. R. (2014). The Darwinian puzzle of declining female happiness. Social Science & Medicine, 120, 252-260.

Levin, B. R., & Rozen, D. E. (2006). Non-inherited antibiotic resistance. Nature Reviews Microbiology, 4(7), 556-562.

Majerus, M. E. (2009). Industrial melanism in the peppered moth, Biston betularia: an excellent teaching example of Darwinian evolution in action. Evolution: Education and Outreach, 2(1), 63-74.

Cherry, K. (2020, February 19). *How confirmation bias works*. Verywell Mind. https://www.verywellmind.com/what-is-a-confirmation-bias-2795024

Gladwell, M. (2008). *Outliers: The Story of Success*. Back Bay Books, Cop.

Glaveski, S. (2021, May 3). *Mindblowing Facts about Your Gut-Brain Connection*. Steve Glaveski. https://medium.com/steveglaveski/mindblowing-facts-about-your-   gut-brain-connection-

1fff90346195#:~:text=The%20vagus%20nerve%20is%20an

Hoomans, J. (2015). *35,000 Decisions: The Great Choices of Strategic Leaders.* Roberts.edu. https://go.roberts.edu/leadingedge/the-great-choices-of-strategic-leaders

InnovateMR. (n.d.). *Imposter Syndrome affects 65% of professionals, new study finds.* Www.prnewswire.com. https://www.prnewswire.com/news-releases/imposter-   syndrome-affects-65-of-professionals-new-study-finds-301295516.html

Li, P., Cheng, Z. yan, & Liu, G. lin. (2020). Availability Bias Causes Misdiagnoses by Physicians: Direct Evidence from a Randomized Controlled Trial. *Internal   Medicine,   59*(24),   3141–3146. https://doi.org/10.2169/internalmedicine.4664-20

Mary Chapin Carpenter , M. C. C. (n.d.). *Dire Straits - The Bug Lyrics | Lyrics.com.* Www.lyrics.com.   Retrieved   July   24,   2023, from https://www.lyrics.com/lyric/4066641/Dire+Straits/The+Bug

Nikolopoulou, K. (2023, February 2). *What Is Negativity Bias? | Definition & Examples.*   Scribbr.   https://www.scribbr.com/research-bias/negativity-bias/#:~:text=Negativity%20bias%20is%20the%20tendency

Penn, A. (2019, November 3). *Narrative Fallacy: 7 Examples of Harmful Storytelling.*   Shortform   Books. https://www.shortform.com/blog/narrative-fallacy/

Satterfield, D. R. (2018, July 26). *Success is 10 percent Inspiration, Leadership in Action.* Leadership in Action. https://www.theleadermaker.com/success-is-10- percent-inspiration/

Seligman, M. E. P. (2018). *Learned optimism.* Nicholas Brealey Publishing.

Seligman, M. E. P., & Csikszentmihalyi, M. (2000). Positive psychology: An   introduction.   *American   Psychologist,   55*(1),   5–14. https://doi.org/10.1037/0003- 066x.55.1.5

Wilczek, F. (2015, September 23). *Einstein's Parable of Quantum Insanity.* Scientific   American.

https://www.scientificamerican.com/article/einstein-s-parable-of- quantum-insanity/

Wolfson, A. (2023, July 24). Oprah Winfrey, now worth an estimated $2.5 billion

Benedetti, F., Lanotte, M., Lopiano, L., & Colloca, L. (2007). When words are painful:aveling the mechanisms of the nocebo effect. Neuroscience, 147(2), -271.

Brody, H., Colloca, L., Miller, F. G., & Ernst, E. (2020). The placebo and nocebo effects: A practical taxonomy for clinicians. Journal of Internal Medicine, 287(2), 119- 135

Colloca, L., & Miller, F. G. (2011). The nocebo effect and its relevance for clinical practice. Psychosomatic Medicine, 73(7), 598-603.

Häuser, W., Hansen, E., & Enck, P. (2012). Nocebo phenomena in medicine: Their relevance in everyday clinical practice. Deutsches Ärzteblatt International, 109(26), 459-465.

Rief, W., & Avorn, J. (2019). The nocebo effect: A narrative review. JAMA, 321(20), 2023-2027.

The Improbable Journey: Jose Altuve From Venezuela Sandlot To World Champion, December 2017, Brad Kyle, Therunnersports.com.

The Power of Writing Down Goals: 42% More Likely to Achieve Success, Banu Akgul, LinkedIn, March 16, 2023.

Angevaren, M., Aufdemkampe, G., Verhaar, H. J., Aleman, A., & Vanhees, L. (2008). Physical activity and enhanced fitness to improve cognitive function in older people without cognitive impairment. The Cochrane Database of Systematic005381.

Beck, A. T. (1979). Cognitive therapy of depression. Guilford Press.

Camic, P. M., Chatterjee, H. J., & Price, L. L. (2013). Creative arts therapies approaches to resilience building among survivors of the London bombings on July 7, 2005. Journal of Traumatic Stress, 26(5), 648-653.

Cohen, S. (2004). Social relationships and health. American Psychologist,

59(8), 676- 684.

Cohen, S., Janicki-Deverts, D., & Miller, G. E. (2015). Psychological stress and disease. JAMA, 313(3), 253-264.

Harris, P. R., Brearley, I., & Sheeran, P. (2018). Emotional resilience and wellbeing: Exploring emotional intelligence and mindfulness in educators and community psychologists. Journal of Public Mental Health, 17(2), 79-99.

Hoge, E. A., Bui, E., Marques, L., Metcalf, C. A., Morris, L. K., Robinaugh, D. J., Worthington, J. J., Pollack, M. H., & Simon, N. M. (2018). Randomized controlled trial meditation for generalized anxiety disorder: on anxiety and stress reactivity. Journal of Clinical Psychiatry, 748), 786-792.

Li, Y., Lv, M. R., Wei, Y., Sun, L., Zhang, J. X., Zhang, H. G., Li, B., Li, L. H., & Yao,

Z. H. (201). Dietary patterns and depression risk: A meta-analysis. Psychiatry Research, 267, 17-26.

Lunstad, J. L., Cacioppo, J. T., &uneberg, J. (2010). Loneliness and social isolation factors for mortality: A meta-analytic review. Perspectives on Psychological Science, 10(2), 227-237.

Pillai, V., Steenburg, L. A., Ciesla, J. A., Roth, T., & Drake, C.

Rahim, M. A. (2017). Managing Conflict in Organizations (5th ed.). Routledge. Folger, J. P., Poole, M. S.,

Cialdini, R. B. (2001). Influence: Science and practice (4th ed.). Boston, MA: Allyn & Bacon.

2.ivers, R. L. (1971). The evolution of reciprocal altruism. The Quarterly Review of Biology, 46(1 35-57.

Fehr, E., & Fischbacher, U. (2003). The nature of human altruism. Nature, 425(6960), 785-791.

Kabat-Zinn, J., Lipworth, L., & Burney, R. (1985). The clinical use of mindfulness meditation for the self-regulation of chronic pain. Journal of Behavioral Medicine, 8(2), 163-190.

Goyal, M., Singh, S., Sibinga, E. M., et al. (2014). Meditation programs for psychological stress and well-being: a systematic review and meta-analysis. JAMA Internal Medicine, 174(3), 357-368.

Black, D. S., O'Reilly, G. A., Olmstead, R., et al. (2015). Mindfulness meditation and improvement in sleep quality and daytime impairment among older adults with sleep disturbances: A randomized clinical trial. JAMA Internal Medicine, 175(4), 494-501.

Ong, J. C., Manber, R., Segal, Z., et al. (2014). A randomized controlled trial of mindfulness meditation for chronic insomnia. Sleep, 37(9), 1553-1563.

Davidson, R. J., Kabat-Zinn, J., Schumacher, J., et al. (2003). Alterations in brain and immune function produced by mindfulness meditation. Psychosomatic Medicine, 65(4), 564-570.

Kuyken, W., Hayes, R., Barrett, B., et al. (2015). Effectiveness and cost-effectiveness of mindfulness-based cognitive therapy compared with maintenance antidepressant treatment in the prevention of depressive relapse or recurrence (PREVENT): a randomised controlled trial. The Lancet, 386(9988), 63-73.

Kabat-Zinn, J. (1994). Wherever You Go, There You Are: Mindfulness Meditation in Everyday Life. Hyperion.

Salzberg, S. (2011). Real Happiness: The Power of Meditation: A 28-Day Program. Workman Publishing Company.

Goleman, D., & Davidson, R.J. (2017). Altered Traits: Science Reveals How Meditation Changes Your Mind, Brain, and Body. Avery.

Harris, D. (2017). 10% Happier: How I Tamed the Voice in My Head, Reduced Stress Without Losing My Edge, and Found Self-Help That Actually Works - A True Story. William Morrow Paperbacks.

Kabat-Zinn, J. (2005). Full Catastrophe Living: Using the Wisdom of Your Body and Mind to Face Stress, Pain, and Illness. Bantam.

Seligman, M. E. P., & Maier, S. F. (1967). Failure to escape traumatic shock. Journal of Experimental Psychology, 74(1), 1-9.

Abramson, L. Y., Seligman, M. E. P., & Teasdale, J. D. (1978). Learned helplessness in humans: Critique and reformulation. Journal of Abnormal Psychology, 87(1), 49-74.

Alloy, L. B., & Abramson, L. Y. (1982). Learned helplessness, depression, and the illusion of control. Journal of Personality and Social Psychology, 42(6), 1114-1126.

Nolen-Hoeksema, S., Girgus, J. S., & Seligman, M. E. P. (1992). Predictors and consequences of childhood depressive symptoms: A 5-year longitudinal study. Journal of Abnormal Psychology, 101(3), 405-422.

Alloy, L. B., Peterson, C., Abramson, L. Y., & Seligman, M. E. P. (1984). Attributional style and the generality of learned helplessness. Journal of Personality and Social Psychology, 46(3), 681-687.